When Your Child Is Sick

2nd edition

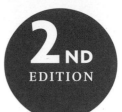

WHEN YOUR CHILD IS SICK

WHAT **YOU** CAN DO TO HELP

PROFESSOR ALF NICHOLSON FRCPI, FRCPCH
AND GRÁINNE O'MALLEY

GILL BOOKS

The information given in this book is intended to support – not replace – discussion with your doctor. Neither the authors nor the publisher can accept legal responsibility for any health problem resulting from the use or misuse of advice described in this book. You should always consult a qualified medical practitioner for specific information on personal health conditions.

Gill Books
Hume Avenue
Park West
Dublin 12
www.gillbooks.ie

Gill Books is an imprint of M.H. Gill & Co.

© Alf Nicholson and Gráinne O'Malley 2016

978 07171 6922 1

Design by Design Image
Illustrations by Andriy Yankovskyy
Indexed by Cliff Murphy
Printed by BZ Graf S.A., Poland

This book is typeset in Agenda and Aptifer Slab.

For permission to reproduce photographs, the authors and publisher gratefully acknowledge the following: © Alamy: 6BL, 24, 25, 28, 30, 48B, 51, 56, 61, 78, 93, 93, 101, 115L, 115B, 123, 126, 132, 138, 148, 150, 151, 156, 160, 162T, 162B, 164, 177, 181B, 193, 210, 246, 257, 270, 271, 279, 283, 287, 290, 297, 300, 304T, 306; Andy Crawford and Steve Gorton © Dorling Kindersley: 106T; © Corbis: 166B; © Getty Images: 14B, 64, 65, 118, 125, 153, 166T, 175, 267B, 269; © Gilles San Martin / www.flickr.com/photos/sanmartin/<http://www.flickr.com/photos/sanmartin/>: 6 (dust mite), 54 (dust mite); © Phototake: 165, 171; Ruth Jenkinson © Dorling Kindersley: 106B; © Science Photo Library: 14C, 96CB, 165, 167, 169, 170, 181T, 303T, 303B, 304B.
Additional images supplied by iStock and Shutterstock.

The authors and publisher have made every effort to trace all copyright holders, but if any have been inadvertently overlooked we would be pleased to make the necessary arrangement at the first opportunity.

The paper used in this book comes from the wood pulp of managed forests. For every tree felled, at least one tree is planted, thereby renewing natural resources.

A CIP catalogue record for this book is available from the British Library.

5 4 3 2 1

I asked many colleagues in paediatrics to review draft manuscripts and I thank them for their time and helpful feedback. Most important, my thanks to my wife, Helen, and to my children, Katie, Mark, Marie Louise and Alfie, for their support while I was writing this book. I dedicate the book to them, to my mother and to my late father.

Alf Nicholson

Many parents read and tested draft material for this book and I am grateful to them and also to our publishers, Gill Books (and especially to Deirdre Nolan, Ruth Mahony and Sarah Liddy), for their help throughout the project. This book is for my family, for their endless patience.

Gráinne O'Malley

The Authors

Alf Nicholson FRCPI, FRCPCH is RCSI Professor of Paediatrics. He is based in Temple Street Children's University Hospital and has over 25 years' experience in the practice of paediatric medicine. He is the National Clinical Lead for Paediatrics in the HSE's National Clinical Programme for Paediatrics and Neonatology and co-dean for basic specialist training in Paediatrics and is responsible for the national programme for junior paediatric trainee doctors in Ireland.

He has worked in Europe and Australia, including the Royal Children's Hospital in Melbourne (the largest paediatric hospital in the southern hemisphere).

He is married with four children.

Gráinne O'Malley is a professional writer with a background in public relations and over 20 years' writing experience. She is a mother of two children.

CONTENTS

Note: We alternate between 'he' and 'she' throughout this book, for balance.

> **IMPORTANT: THE INFORMATION IN THIS BOOK IS NOT INTENDED AS A SUBSTITUTE FOR YOUR OWN DOCTOR. ALWAYS CONSULT YOUR DOCTOR IF THERE IS ANY CAUSE FOR CONCERN.**

Preface

When I wrote the first edition of *When Your Child Is Sick*, I was bothered that large numbers of children were visiting the doctor or hospital more frequently than in the past. Hospitalisation rates were high and this had to be traumatic for families. It seemed to me that parents were deeply anxious and had lost some confidence in handling their own children's illnesses. There were many reasons for this anxiety, not least the confusion of expertise across the internet.

In writing this second edition, I remain guided by these concerns. Our hospitals and doctors' surgeries are still unnecessarily full. Thankfully, however, there is now a consensus in national health bodies: hospitals should be for our sickest children, but in general healthcare should be carried out as close to home as possible.

After all, children growing up today are one of the healthiest generations ever. Thanks to better living standards and vaccination, many 'killer' infectious diseases have disappeared. However, we are now seeing a rise in lifestyle-related diseases, such as obesity, asthma and allergies. The good news is that many of these can be managed by an experienced parent in the home – so long as the parent knows when to call for help.

I believe that we need to remind ourselves what is normal when a child is sick. As most doctors know:

- The same ailments crop up time and again – some 20 ailments, in fact.
- What is likely to be wrong is usually very minor.
- Most of the time, a child can be treated at home by the parent.

In the new edition of *When Your Child Is Sick*, I have reflected on what has changed in child health in the seven years since the first edition was published and what is happening now in medicine in Europe and North America. I have made significant additions to the chapters on allergy, obesity and hyperactivity – areas that continue to cause grief for many parents – and have considered the most advanced thinking. I have also expanded the chapter on complementary health remedies to help parents find their way safely through the many options available. I have advised some caution but, throughout the book, where a natural product has shown itself in trials to be effective and safe, I have recommended it.

When Your Child Is Sick works because it can be easily used by any parent or carer. It's not simply an aid to understanding what is wrong – it gets to the heart of each ailment, giving you a picture of what's going on and how you can prevent a recurrence. And when illness strikes, the Red Alert system helps you find answers fast. At a glance, you can learn how to treat it at home and the danger signs that need a call for help.

When Your Child Is Sick also keeps the parents' perspective uppermost at all times. As experienced parents, my co-author, Gráinne O'Malley, and I appreciate the great concerns that families face when a child gets sick. Everything in the book is aimed at answering these concerns and every piece of information is based on researched medical evidence.

There are, in the main, 20 reasons why children are taken to the doctor. *When Your Child Is Sick* is built around these 20 ailments and is designed to answer every parent's health worry: 'Is this normal?'

I wrote this new edition because I believe that parents can, and want to, play a larger role in making their sick children better. I also hope that it will go some way towards helping our hard-pressed medical profession. It is not a substitute for your doctor, but an informed and sensible parent is a tremendous ally for any doctor.

Professor Alf Nicholson, FRCPI, FRCPCH

Section 1
The Top 20 Children's Ailments

KNOW HOW TO TREAT YOUR CHILD AT HOME –
AND WHEN TO CALL THE DOCTOR

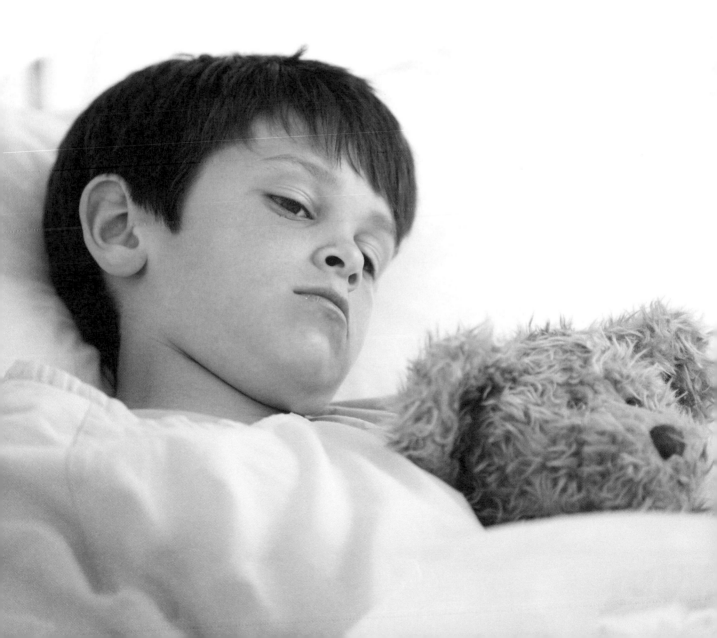

Chapter 1

Asthma

'He seems to get breathless very easily and now he's started coughing at night. Every time he gets a cold it takes ages for him to get over it. Maybe he's just prone to chest infections? He does eventually get better on antibiotics but then it all comes back after a few weeks. Please don't tell me it's asthma.'

Inhalers Everywhere

School classrooms are awash with inhalers these days, but are we overreacting? Not if you consider that until recently 5 per cent of children in developed countries had asthma; today up to 20 per cent do. That has to be worrying.

We need to be careful with asthma because a severe attack can be fatal. But with modern asthma therapy your child should be able to live a normal life – and play sports without coughing and wheezing. Remember that:

- Asthma is the **temporary** narrowing of the airways in the lungs.
- An asthma attack usually coincides with a viral infection.
- You can control asthma, especially if you use inhalers correctly.
- Most children outgrow it before their teens.

You should not be afraid of, or ignore, the diagnosis.

Is It Asthma?

The answer is rarely easy or quick. But I will always suspect it when parents report regular coughing – a cough that won't go away. I look for:

- Dry coughing (no mucus) at night and early morning.
- Wheezing (high-pitched, whistling sounds) when breathing out.
- Shortness of breath or coughing when exercising.
- Regular chest tightness.
- Other allergic conditions such as eczema or hay fever.
- A likely trigger, such as a chest infection or smoke.

It will all tend to disturb sleep and day-to-day life. Your child may be prone to chest infections and have coughing problems every time he gets one – mainly when lying down. He may even have a puffed-out chest, like a pigeon (he's not emptying his lungs completely and air is trapped in the tiny air sacs). Wheezing is common – but not every asthmatic child wheezes.

There's no 'gold standard' test, I'm afraid, for asthma with small children. Your child will be diagnosed from his medical history and – to a large extent – from the symptoms you report as the parent. At age six, we can test lung function with laboratory tests. Allergy skin-prick tests are popular, but they won't confirm asthma.

Or Something Else?

We cannot always assume that asthma is the cause.

PROBLEMS THAT MIMIC ASTHMA

Main problems	Main symptoms
Viral wheezing	Your child wheezes when he catches a viral infection. Most grow out of it before they start school.
Inhaled object	Your child is well, then suddenly has a dramatic wheeze.
Cystic fibrosis	Your child is not gaining much weight (despite good appetite) and he may have polyps in the nose.
Habit cough	Your child has a regular, barking cough (like a seal) that always disappears when sleeping.

With most of these, asthma inhalers will not seem to help. It may not be asthma if the coughing dates from birth or if he is sickly.

OUR BREATHING SYSTEM

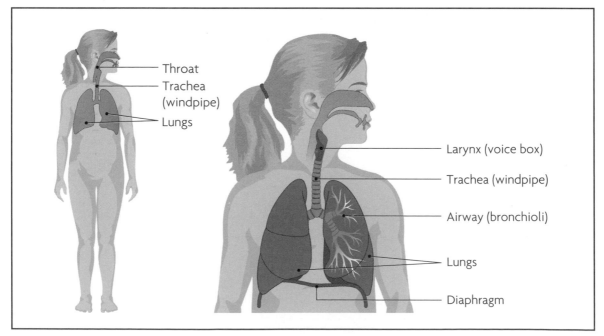

Throat
Trachea (windpipe)
Lungs

Larynx (voice box)
Trachea (windpipe)
Airway (bronchioli)
Lungs
Diaphragm

Asthma Triggers

A lot of triggers can set off an asthma attack. Your child will have his own favourites. It may be surprising to find that food is not a common asthma trigger. In fact, the most likely trigger for his asthma will be inhaled.

- Indoor allergens such as pet fur, damp moulds (damp houses can cause asthma).
- Outdoor allergens such as pollen from trees, grass and weeds.
- Exercise.
- Chest infections.
- Air pollutants such as tobacco smoke, fumes and aerosol sprays.
- Stress and extreme emotions.
- Cold, dry air.
- Medicines (e.g. aspirin).
- The house dust mite. (By far the biggest trigger; it loves our overheated houses.)

The Hygiene Hypothesis

What's behind the rise and rise of asthma? Dr David Strachan's 'hygiene hypothesis' is now widely accepted and new evidence from 2014 studies has reinforced it. It holds that exposure to dirty environments reduces the risk of allergic disease. In the past, we got used to infections, damp and dust when we lived (or survived) ten to a cottage – with our animals. These days we are cosseted with cleanliness from birth and are less exposed to bacteria. So our immune systems have changed and we are less able to handle allergens. They set off more extreme reactions. Worse, our houses are now energy-efficient boxes that seal us in with them.

There is something to be said for the old approach after all. Get your baby outside in all weathers (except for fog) as long as he is wrapped up well. Get toddlers' hands a little dirty. Get them out in the garden or down to the farm and expose them to certain bacteria. Cocooning them in houses and crèches – those sealed, overheated environments – certainly does not help asthma.

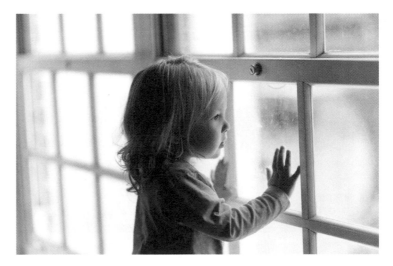

WHEN BREATHING GOES WRONG

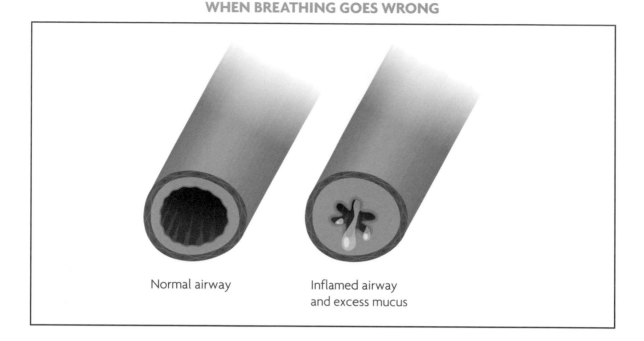

Normal airway

Inflamed airway
and excess mucus

Asthma Medication

The biggest concern with asthma is to keep the lungs from getting too inflamed. Most asthma medication is sucked into the airways and he will use one (or both) types of inhaler: relievers and preventers. Preventers are steroids; relievers are not. For information on how to use inhalers, see pages 14–15.

RELIEVERS are enough if he is **occasionally** wheezy. They open up his airways when he has breathing problems – or before strenuous exercise.

The standard inhaler contains salbutamol and your child inhales it directly into the lungs (in fact, most of it is swallowed and less than 30 per cent actually gets into the lungs, but that is more than enough). It usually works within minutes, relieving for about four hours. This is a bronchodilator; the chemical acts on the beta2 receptors in the airways to open them. It is very safe and only has side effects (a faster heartbeat and hand tremor) if he takes a very high dose.

Sometimes the asthma simply will not ease and then he needs a short, sharp dose of oral steroids for a few days. These will not work instantly – it takes over four hours – but they are powerful and just as effective as any steroid given on a drip. They should be used sparingly.

PREVENTERS If asthma is a **regular** problem, your child will need a preventer too. This aims to keep the lungs healthy by preventing inflammation. He uses the reliever as well if he needs it.

When the child uses a preventer (e.g. beclamethazone or budesonide), he inhales corticosteroids twice a day. The average dose is small and is quite safe. If that is not controlling the asthma, I would advise a combination inhaler — the next-step treatment. This is a mix of inhaled corticosteroid and a longer-acting salbutamol.

There is also a leukotriene modifier, which is newer and can help children over two years old who have regular asthma. It changes the chemistry in the airways and helps to keep them open. Children like it because it is easy to take (at bedtime) and many parents like it because it is not a steroid. It is effective, but may occasionally cause nightmares.

Are You in Control?

I get concerned about asthma control when:

- A child regularly forgets to take his inhaler.
- More than two courses of steroids were prescribed in the past year.
- There have been visits to hospital with a severe wheeze.
- A child has been admitted to hospital.
- Antibiotics are frequently prescribed.
- There are regular visits to the family doctor.
- The parents are lukewarm about using asthma drugs.

Complacency is a real problem: 'He's better so I stopped the medication.'

Home Treatment: Asthma

A lot of controlling asthma is down to the parent. You really need to know your child's symptoms intimately, so you can spot the warning signs. Your aim is to get in early (with the **minimum** of drugs) so that he can lead a normal life with few or no coughing symptoms.

There should be no reason to restrict his lifestyle. I would hate to see a child missing school or sports because of asthma.

Controlling Asthma

- **Write up an Asthma Plan** with your doctor. This is the daily record of medication your child uses and any asthma symptoms. It should include a rescue plan for times when his asthma is more severe (e.g. the dosage automatically increases depending on his peak flow measurements).

- **Use a peak flow meter** (if your child is over six and gets regular attacks) to see how healthy the lungs are. Use it twice a day as routine and more often if there are problems.

- **Learn to use his inhalers** and show anyone who cares for him (see pages 14–15). Use a spacer with the inhaler (without it, less than 5 per cent gets into the lungs, but with it he'll get over 20 per cent; and for most asthma they are as good as a nebuliser). Use an aerochamber spacer until age three, then switch to a large-volume spacer. Wash the spacer twice a month and drip dry it.

- **A reliever inhaler** is enough for most children and, ideally, they should need very little or none. Give it as soon as symptoms start. But when he gets a chest infection, it is a good idea to give more. Use it also before your child is exposed to one of his asthma triggers (such as exercise or animals). Keep spares in the car, school or crèche.

- **If your child has regular asthma**, he will also need to use a preventer every day. Don't stop using it when his asthma calms down, or it will come back. He should not be on a preventer or a combination inhaler unless the asthma is chronic.

- **Don't use cough medicines** to treat a cough. A drink of water will be just as effective.

- **Don't change diet**, as food (including milk) is almost certainly not causing the asthma. There is no 'asthma diet'.

- **Let him play outdoors** as much as possible and open your windows daily, unless the pollen count is high.

- **Try to avoid his asthma trigger.** If animal fur sets it off, you may have to reconsider your pets or at least keep them outside – and never let them in your child's bedroom. If damp mould is a trigger, be wary of damp houses, building sites or house renovations. Damp spores are often released into the air when old walls are opened up.

- **Don't smoke near your child** as this can trigger asthma, and make sure he does not start himself. (If you are a smoker, it will make things difficult.)

- **Try to avoid** wood-burning stoves, sprays and other air pollutants.

- **Reduce house dust mite** as far as you can:
    - The key is ventilation. Open your windows and install trickle vents if you have double glazing.
    - Do not have carpets or rugs in the bedroom.

- Use special dust-proof covers on the mattress and pillows.
- Wash bedding and mattress covers weekly at a high temperature (at least 54°C is needed to kill the mites) and dry on a hot cycle.
- Damp dust all bedroom surfaces weekly.
- Use washable curtains on the bedroom windows.
- Have washable soft toys only and wash them weekly.
- Using a vacuum with a HEPA filter will not help (it only works for airborne allergens, not mites). Air cleaning sprays don't get rid of dust mites or their droppings.

- **Immunotherapy** is a growing but generally untried field. It has tested quite well with hay fever, but there has been no success yet with asthma.
- **Buteyko** and other breathing training techniques help some children and may be worth trying.
- **He does not need an annual flu vaccine**, unless his asthma is severe.
- **If you are not in control** make sure you're using the inhalers correctly. Are you spotting the warning signs and using the inhalers early enough? Are you increasing the dosage when he needs it? Is he on the right inhaler? Talk to your doctor if control is still a problem.

And be careful when your child reaches adolescence. He risks becoming complacent and – out of sight – symptoms can silently creep up on you all.

When He Has an Asthma Attack

- **Use the normal reliever** with the spacer. Give up to ten puffs.
- **Sit him upright** to help breathing, piling pillows behind him.
- **Using steroid tablets** may have some merit, if you have experience with them. But they will take several hours to take effect.
- **Open the window** to change the air.
- **Reassure your child.** Tell him he will be better soon. Turn the light on, try a favourite drink, a light massage – whatever will help to relax him, as anxiety can make things worse.
- **But do not give him anything with a sedative;** this could suppress the natural respiratory drive and be dangerous.
- **Encourage slow, deep breathing;** If he is a frequent sufferer, it may be worth learning a simple breathing exercise.
- **Stay close** to him all the time.
- **Get help** if he's not responding (see Red Alert, page 17). Be quick to get help with an asthma attack.

Is It Hay Fever?

If your child has asthma, he is quite likely to get hay fever too because the nose and lungs are all part of the same breathing system. Hay fever (allergic rhinitis) is an allergic reaction around the nose and eyelids. He will have two or more of these symptoms:

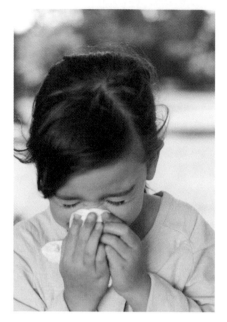

- He is always sniffling and blowing his nose. But the mucus is clear and watery.
- His nose itches a lot. He may rub the tip of it with his palm, pushing upwards in the 'allergic salute'.
- He has regular sneezing fits that go on and on.
- His eyes are watery and itch.
- He may breathe through his mouth.

He will be clear for months, and then it comes back. This is because the allergy is usually to tree pollens in early spring, and grass pollens in late spring and early summer. It will be an inhaled problem and in some cases it can be a reaction to house dust mites or animal dander. The timing is very relevant. When he is exposed to the allergen, symptoms will start quickly – in minutes – and last for hours.

Home Treatment: Hay Fever

Reactions to treatment will vary, depending on the child, but most can find some relief.

- **When pollen counts are high**, keep windows closed and limit his time outdoors if he has hay fever. Avoid contact with pollen if you can. That means avoiding compost piles, hay, mown grass, raked leaves or any pollinating plants. Daily baths can help.
- **If dander or house dust mites are the trigger**, try to minimise exposure (see under Controlling Asthma, page 10).
- **Try antihistamines first.** They are good at tackling all the sneezing and itching and will help the eye problems too. (The newer ones will not make the child feel drowsy.) But they will not do a lot for a blocked nose.
- **If his nose is blocked**, a nasal decongestant will help (it reduces blood supply to the nose). It can be used with antihistamines.

➕ **Salt water sprays and saline drops** may help to relieve symptoms with some children. Butterbur is sometimes used as a natural alternative to antihistamines, but children should only use it under medical supervision. Nasal steroids work best, but are expensive, slow to act and the effects are short lived (nose drops are kinder to his nose than sprays). They do not help itching, so he may also need antihistamines.

➕ **If nothing works,** you could consider immunotherapy, which has had some success. But you must start treatment before the pollen season begins and ideally continue it for three years.

Is It Sinusitis?

This is sometimes confused with hay fever, so it is worth clearing things up a little. Sinusitis is inflammation of the sinuses (the air-filled tubes around the nose) caused by an infection. When it is bad, he will usually have:

➕ A temperature and a headache.

➕ A stuffed nose, but constantly dripping mucus that is thick and yellowish.

➕ Coughing during the day (but no wheeze).

➕ Some swelling around his face or eyelids.

➕ Loss of smell and taste.

It starts like a cold, but his nose will stream for days on end – even up to a month. He will probably disgust you all by snorting back the mucus or by swallowing the revolting stuff.

Home Treatment: Sinusitis

➕ **Antibiotics are needed** as sinusitis is a bacterial infection; decongestants will not be very useful for the blocked nose, but steam can help to clear it. Try inhaling steam under a towel or sit him in the bathroom with the hot taps on – but be careful with hot water!

➕ **Saline drops** are a good idea for the first few days, to clean the nasal passages.

➕ **Neti pots, bulb syringes** and other nasal irrigation devices (to rinse out the sinuses) have been popular but now carry health warnings. If not used properly, there is a risk of serious infection.

➕ **Give him paracetamol** to relieve any pain or temperature.

➕ **Nasal steroids** are not advised unless sinusitis is a regular problem.

How to Use Asthma Inhalers

For smaller children, using a spacer or Aerochamber mask with the inhaler is usually an easier way of getting the medicine into the lungs. Timing is less of an issue, as the medicine collects in the chamber until it is breathed in. But turbohalers should only be used on children over six years of age.

When you first use an inhaler, explain to your child how it is going to work. Let him feel it, shake it or pretend to use it on a toy first.

Inhaler with Volumatic Spacer

- Remove the cap.
- Shake the inhaler and insert it in the spacer.
- Put the spacer mouthpiece in his mouth.
- He should breathe in and out, slowly and gently. You should hear a clicking noise (as the valve opens and closes).
- Once there is a breathing pattern, press the inhaler canister once (keeping the inhaler in the same position). He should continue breathing several more times, but deeper breathing.

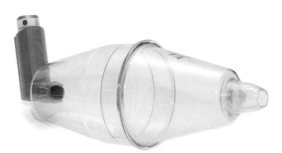

Inhaler with volumatic spacer

- Remove the mouthpiece from his mouth. Wait about 30 seconds, then repeat the dose.
- The first time you use the inhaler (or if you have not used it for two weeks), you need to prime it. Shake it and spray it into the air a few times, then use as normal.

Inhaler with Aerochamber

- Remove the inhaler cap.
- Make sure the mask is fitted on snugly. Flexible masks seem to create a better seal than rigid masks.
- Insert the inhaler (upright) into the aerochamber.
- Holding the aerochamber and inhaler, shake everything two or three times.

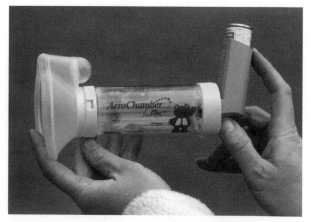

Inhaler with aerochamber

- Place the facemask so that it covers his mouth and nose (creating a seal with his face).
- Press the inhaler canister once. Hold the mask over his face for up to six breaths, or as long as he will tolerate it.
- Repeat the dose if necessary.

He may object to a mask on his face, but if you hold the mask even a **little** away from his face the dose will be markedly less. You can also give him the medication while he is asleep.

Turbohaler

- Unscrew and remove the white cover.
- Hold the inhaler upright. Twist the coloured base as far as it will go in both directions until you hear a clicking sound. Now it is loaded and ready to use.
- Get him to breathe out (away from the mouthpiece).
- Hold the mouthpiece in his mouth and ask him to breathe in as deeply as possible.

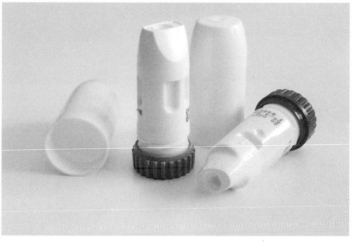

Turbohaler

- Remove the turbohaler and let him breathe out.
- Repeat for a second dose.
- Always replace the white cover.
- The dose counter will change from a white background to a red one when the number 20 shows in the window. When the 0 on the red background reaches the middle of the window, the inhaler is empty.

Before you use a new turbohaler for the first time, follow these instructions but **repeat** the second step. This primes it.

Source: Based on guidelines from the National Respiratory Training Centre.

Q&A

Q **I'm very reluctant to keep dosing such a small child with chemicals. Surely they can't be good for him in the long term? I'd prefer more natural remedies.**

A I can sympathise. Nobody likes to give any child drugs over a long period and many parents try therapies such as acupuncture, herbal medicines, omega 3 fatty acids and homeopathy. But if your child has asthma, you are not likely to find that they control the problem. Certainly the research does not support it.

So far, anti-inflammatory drugs have proved the best way of keeping your asthmatic child safe. The trick is to find the minimal dose that will keep his asthma under control. In fact, the amount of steroids he inhales with his preventer is tiny (some 10 per cent goes straight into his airways), and the side effects really are negligible. A high dose would certainly be a problem because he could absorb small amounts of steroid into his body. But he would need to be taking 800 micrograms a day to be at risk of this. The average daily dose in his preventer is only 200 micrograms. You should, however, try to limit the steroid tablets he takes as over-use can have long-term effects.

Don't undervalue asthma inhalers. I regularly see children who missed out on school and normal activities for years and whose lives have been transformed by them. They really are quite remarkable for those children who need them.

Q **Milk seems to make him wheeze, so I've started to cut out dairy products. Is it asthma and will this help?**

A Food does not cause asthma – we simply have not managed to nail any link to it. Nor has milk been proven to cause excessive mucus, though this is a popular belief. You will find children with food allergies who have asthma, but they are more likely to have a general allergic tendency. The milk–mucus theory continues, although a study of 3,000 pre-school children in the Netherlands found that those who consumed the **most** products containing milk had a reduced risk of developing asthma. Some foods can certainly make asthma worse, for example drinking large quantities of fructose-sweetened drinks. By all means, cut out your child's sweetened drinks, but don't reduce his milk.

Q **We smoke outside, away from our children, so what's the problem?**

A Cigarette smoke makes asthma coughing worse. Smoking outside the house is not the answer, I'm afraid, as the smoke is still present on your clothes and in your hair. When you return inside, this smoke diffuses into the atmosphere and your child breathes it in. It's also worth knowing that children of parents who smoke are about twice as likely to develop asthma.

Q Will he grow out of his asthma?

A Parents expect a definitive 'yes' to this question – and generally children do outgrow asthma. After all, 20 per cent of children have asthma while only 5 per cent of adults do. The best long-term studies of asthma found that those with mild asthma usually outgrew it. But if his asthma is severe and persistent as a child, he is less likely to outgrow it. Try to keep him away from smoking when he is an adolescent, as it really plays havoc with asthma.

Babies Who Wheeze

🐻 Doctors are slow to diagnose asthma – not until your child is two years old. 'Wheezy babies' are not unusual. Many wheeze every time they get a viral infection (or when teething) and babies of smoking mothers are especially prone to it. But it is not a sign of asthma and a reliever may have little effect.

🐻 Will your wheezy baby go on to develop asthma? It is often hard to predict, but the chances are higher if he also has eczema or other allergic symptoms and if his wheezing eases when you use an inhaler.

Red Alert

Be quick to get help with an asthma attack.

CALL A DOCTOR OR HOSPITAL **IMMEDIATELY** IF:

✚ The breathing is fast and shallow.

✚ He is so breathless that he cannot complete a sentence when he talks.

✚ He is constantly coughing.

✚ His colour changes. If his lips seem blue, go straight to a hospital.

✚ Trust your instincts. If it feels dramatically wrong, it probably is.

Chapter 2
Colic

'For the first few weeks, she was a very sunny little baby, feeding and sleeping quite easily. We felt so lucky. But now she's like a different child. She cries so much, most of all in the evening, and nothing I do seems to console her. She really seems to be in such pain, it can't simply be colic.'

When the 'Dream Baby' Turns

Every baby cries, but is it normal when your dream baby turns into a screamer overnight? For quite a large number of babies (up to one in four) it can be.

Colic is very real, very difficult to manage and it will push your own limits. Doctors are fascinated by colic, but I have huge sympathy for anyone who has to live with it every day. If it is any reassurance:

- A child with colic is usually perfectly healthy.
- No matter how bad it is, it should stop within four months.
- Drugs and changes in formula have virtually no role to play.
- While there's no single remedy, you can help your baby.

You will need support with this one; someone to share the job and keep you sane for those few weeks; someone to remind you that your baby will bounce back soon, none the worse for wear. But make sure it is colic first.

Why Babies Cry (Normally)

If only babies could talk. But they communicate by crying and at first it is expressive – baby is bothered and it is one loud universal shout. By three months old, her central nervous system has matured a little and her crying starts to communicate. Now when baby is bothered, she is calling you.

Do babies always cry because something is wrong? Yes; they are not simply manipulating you – that's the toddler's job! But what is wrong may be as basic as tiredness or wanting a cuddle. Normal babies have their own crying style – some cry more (and louder) than others and are slower to soothe.

Most babies follow the same crying pattern, whatever culture they live in or its attitude to rearing children. There is usually a crying 'peak' around four to six weeks old and then it all eases off around eight to 12 weeks – a little earlier if baby is bottle-fed. That's normal.

Colic Crying

What is not so normal is colic or 'excessive' crying. Your colic baby will cry more intensely and at a higher pitch than 'normal' crying and will sound as if she is in pain. She may also cry for longer – up to an hour at a time – and will resist most of your efforts to soothe her, including feeding. Her tiny fists may clench, legs may stiffen and she may grimace. She may also throw up milk or be windy.

If it is bad, she may arch her back.

This crying tyrant will typically show up at around two weeks old and sweeten again at about four months. The bouts of colic will usually start and end for no obvious reason. Unfortunately for you, it is often in the evening when you are already worn out.

If you are used to an ordered life, the mayhem she causes can be especially hard to take. But do remember: she's crying because she's bothered and she has absolutely no idea what may be wrong.

Is It Colic?

Colic is never a quick diagnosis. The Wessel Rule of Threes is the system traditionally used by doctors: if your baby cries for more than three hours a day for more than three days a week for three weeks, she has colic. But what parent with a screaming baby will wait that long?

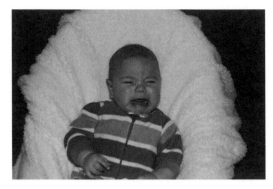

- I suspect colic if your baby has cried intensely for three hours a day for three days of the past week – if there is no other cause.
- I look for typical 'colic crying' symptoms.
- Tests are rarely needed.

Or Something Else?

The vast majority of babies who cry excessively have colic. But when your baby is screaming hard and has a temperature or other symptoms, we want to rule out a serious bacterial infection – such as meningitis, septicaemia or a urinary tract infection (see page 92).

There are other medical problems that can mimic colic but they are actually quite rare.

PROBLEMS THAT MIMIC COLIC

Problem	How likely?
Cow's milk protein allergy	Less than 5 per cent of colicky infants
Effects of drugs the mother is taking	A growing problem
Reflux from the oesophagus	Rare
Lactose intolerance	Rare

If you are breastfeeding and taking drugs, there may be a link. Some mother's medications (especially drugs for anxiety and depression) can cause symptoms in a baby that are very like colic. Clues that point to something other than colic are a **very** high-pitched cry with an arched back, a colic that does not happen mainly in the evening, crying that starts at around three months of age or crying that increases dramatically when you change from breast to formula feeding.

The Inside Track

Surprisingly, though we have been studying colic for years, it is still a bit of an enigma. No one has yet shown a single cause (or a single cure) for it.

About a third of colicky babies will improve on treatment. But it may not be the same treatment and the crying may ease but not stop altogether. Which points the finger at more than one cause. Most studies have now narrowed them down to any (or a mix) of three:

* The windy gut.
* The demanding temperament.
* The feeding theory.

A 'windy gut' is often blamed, though it still hasn't been proved, and very few colicky babies cry because of wind. But tests go on. It's thought that the tiny digestive system is still working out how to release wind. Babies do create more gas in the colon during their first three months because they are not too good at absorbing lactose. But any evidence that this extra gas causes colic is really very weak. Of course, raucous crying and gulping will really fill her with air and then you have a vicious circle. There is some evidence that **how** you feed your baby can help.

The idea of the 'demanding baby' is gathering support. Your colicky baby's only thought for the first weeks is sheer survival (after leaving the cosy womb). Then she tries to make sense of her new world and she may be more sensitive (or downright demanding) than others. Other factors include sensitivity to noise, fatigue, too little or too much attention. When something distresses your child, her instinct is to keep shouting. It's her 'white noise' to shut it all out and it may take a lot to calm her because she is really very new to the whole business. Of course, if your baby is stressed it will stress you and one feeds off the other.

The 'feeding theory' (what she is eating) has some basis too. Maybe you are putting a bottle in her mouth every time she cries? Babies are generally self-regulating and spew out surplus milk, but if she is bothered and sucky she may overfeed. A tiny minority of

+ Let her suck on a dummy (if nothing else it can distract her).

+ Use the traditional 'colic carry'. Lie her, face down, over your lap on your forearm, to increase pressure on her stomach.

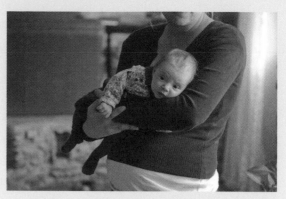

Holding your baby in the 'colic carry' increases pressure on the stomach and can help with colic

- **Over-stimulation can make it all worse,** so less is probably best. I know colic parents who take to bed every evening with a book and a swaddled baby!

- **Don't expect a miracle cure** and be wary of anyone who offers one. Find your own routine and a lot of patience. It will get better.

Q&A

Q I've been told that it's just a question of routines. If I keep her to a strict feeding and sleeping routine, will it make a difference?

A Some parents swear by rigorous routines of sleeping and feeding, but they may not be to everyone's taste and are too regimented for small babies. I am not an advocate of an approach that attempts to train a baby to 'cry it out'.

Q Is she in pain when she gets a colic attack?

A More likely she is very bothered – hungry, overtired or over-stimulated – and crying is her only way of expressing it. If too much wind is the problem, then she may feel very uncomfortable but not in extreme pain.

Q But animals get colic, don't they, and it's serious?

A Colic in animals (mainly horses) is very different from colic in humans. They are herbivores and their digestive system is built to deal with cellulose from grass. They also ferment food in their colon, not in the stomach like us. Sometimes excess methane gas can be trapped in an animal's colon and it is very dangerous if not released. Luckily, we don't eat grass and we don't produce methane gas. Colic in humans is not dangerous.

Q I'm breastfeeding. Could I be the problem? Maybe the food I'm eating is affecting her through my milk. Should I switch to bottle-feeding just in case?

A Please do not stop breastfeeding. It is good for your baby and there is really no evidence that a switch will help. Colic happens to breastfed and bottle-fed babies equally. There is some evidence, though, that a breastfeeding mother can pass allergies to her child. So you might try cutting out high allergens such as nuts, eggs and seafood from your own diet.

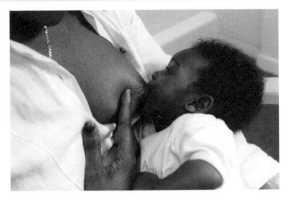

Q Are there any drugs or herbal remedies I can use?

A No colic drug or drop has yet been proved in tests to be safe and effective. This includes lactase enzyme drops, gripe water, simethicone, dicyclomine and methylscopolamine. Dicyclomine did reduce colic crying but has been withdrawn for small babies because of bad side effects. Methylscopolamine is neither safe nor effective for babies with colic. Other drugs can contain alcohol.

Some herbs are used for colic because they reduce spasm – chamomile, fennel seed and lemon balm. In one controlled trial, herbal tea made from these herbs and liquorice was shown to reduce crying considerably. Studies of homeopathic treatments for colic found they were no more effective than placebo pills.

Q Is it caused by reflux and acid in the stomach? If so, what can I do?

A It used to be fashionable to blame colic on acid reflux from the stomach. In reflux, which is a very real condition for some babies, a weak muscle in the oesophagus causes milk and acid to come back up and cause pain. Ask your doctor to rule it out, but remember that it is less likely to be the cause of your baby's distress. Anti-reflux medicines are rarely helpful with colic, unless there is vomiting.

Q Some people say the colic is caused by an imbalance of bacteria in the gut and recommend probiotics. Should I try them?

A Probiotics are simply friendly bacteria and are used in an attempt to re-balance the bacteria in a baby's gut. They have been tried with some success.

Q **I'm very confused. Some people say to let her cry, others say I should pick her up at once.**

A Don't simply ignore a crying baby, but by all means use your common sense. Short crying episodes can be fine, as long as the crying is not high-pitched or too distressed. There is no need to lie awake waiting for the first cry, nor should you rush to pick her up at the first whimper. In fact, constantly picking your baby up can over-stimulate her. When the whimper becomes distressed crying, she needs you to comfort her. I am uneasy with 'controlled crying' techniques for babies under six months.

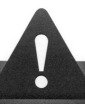

Red Alert

If it is all getting on top of you, you need to visit your doctor. Doctors take the problem of colic very seriously.

CALL A DOCTOR AT ONCE IF YOUR CHILD IS:

- Under three months old and also has a temperature.
- Over three months and also has a temperature with other symptoms (see page 92).
- Very pale, screaming and has blood in her stools (it could be a bowel problem called intussusception).

Please get help now if you worry that your child may get hurt because of you – or your partner's – distress.

Chapter 3

Chest Infection

'It started with a blocked nose and a bit of a cold. But now he has a temperature and a nasty cough and his breathing is very chesty. I'm wondering if the infection has gone down into his chest. Should he have antibiotics?'

In General

Most parents call them chest infections. Doctors call them respiratory illnesses. When you consult your doctor about a 'chest infection', it's not a simple matter of prescribing antibiotics. You are both looking at a fistful of possibilities and the answer may not even lie in your child's chest. (Have you noticed that the symptoms are a little different each time?)

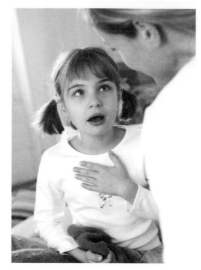

- Over 90 per cent of respiratory infections are viral and **do not need** antibiotics, even if they drag on (the coughing can last up to three weeks). Unless a bacterial infection joins in and makes things worse.

- As a rule of thumb, if your child has a temperature, is breathing quickly and it is an effort, it's most likely an infection in the chest. If your child is sniffling and sneezing, it's not.

- Quite often the 'cough that won't go away' is asthma.

- Watch out for worsening. Most chest infections will self-cure, but sometimes the virus spreads down the lungs (or mucus gets infected by bacteria). (See Red Alert, page 37.)

Is It a Common Cold?

Common colds are upper respiratory infections in the nose and throat.

- The child is sniffling and sneezing.
- He may cough a little and have a sore throat.
- He may have a mild temperature.
- Apart from a little grumpiness, he will go about his business.

All that coughing and sneezing is an effort to expel a virus (most often a rhinovirus). After a day or two and with **no help** it will be gone. As the child grows, the immune system will toughen and produce antibodies to many of the viruses. But he won't outgrow colds because the prevalent virus in your area is (very cleverly) always changing.

THE SYMPTOMS OF A COLD

Nasal congestion

Runny nose

Sore throat

Home Treatment: Cold

A common cold self-cures. It is all helped along by a little tender loving care.

- **Make him cosy** and soothe him with hot drinks (most cold 'remedies' simply do this).
- **If his nose is blocked**, menthol drops on his pyjamas (or menthol inhaling if he is older) can help.
- **A little paracetamol** can help him to sleep if he is restless.
- **Decongestants** (antihistamine) do not help children. Studies have found that they work no better for colds than a placebo.
- **Antibiotics** are never needed for colds or upper respiratory infections.
- **Cold remedies** treat the symptoms, but don't cure colds. Cough suppressants and probiotics have little effect, but recent evidence shows that traditional honey does help. But never give honey to babies under one year, because of infantile botulism.
- **Vitamins** won't prevent (but they may shorten) a cold.
- **Chest clapping** (chest physio), to release mucus from the lungs, has no effect on colds.
- **He is okay to go to school**, unless he is very miserable. The virus is probably around the school already.

Is It Flu or Influenza?

Flu – or influenza – is quite another matter:

- Your child simply won't get up.
- There will be a temperature, usually over 39°C.
- His head will be sore and he will ache all over.
- He may have a dry cough.
- He will have no interest whatsoever in food or playing.

Influenza viruses cause flu and your school-going child is most likely to catch it.

Each winter a different strain of virus does the rounds and this year's vaccine will be developed for this year's virus. When there is a sizeable change in the circulating strain of virus, you get an epidemic or (luckily more rarely) a worldwide pandemic.

Influenza will normally self-cure but it may take over a week.

Home Treatment: Flu

- **Talk to your doctor** and make sure it is influenza.
- **Lower his temperature** with ibuprofen or paracetamol.
- **Cool his body** if need be, by stripping him down to his vest. Try sponging him with a facecloth and lukewarm (not cold!) water.
- **Give him regular (but small) sips of water.** Ice pops can go down easily too.
- **Watch him** for other symptoms and for a temperature rise.
- **Antibiotics** are not needed as the infection is viral.
- **Keep him off school** and in bed until his temperature is normal and he feels much better. It can take five days or more.

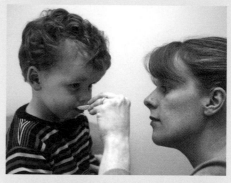

Lower your child's high temperature with ibuprofen or paracetamol

Most children don't need a flu vaccine, but if he has health problems he should have it every autumn.

Is It Bronchiolitis?

Bronchiolitis is mainly a baby infection and a real pest — nearly a third of all babies will develop it before their first birthday. There are epidemics every year in the colder months.

- It starts like a cold, with a temperature, runny nose and cough.
- Then the cough gets worse. He may wheeze too.
- Then his breathing gets faster than normal and becomes an effort.
- He may find it hard to feed properly because he cannot breathe.
- He may even frighten you with short pauses in his breathing.

If your doctor examines his lungs, they will squeak and crackle. It is a viral infection (usually a virus known as RSV) which has spread into the lungs — down into the tiniest air passages, the bronchi and bronchioli. These have become swollen and this makes it more difficult for your baby to breathe. Most babies get better within two weeks, although the cough can take longer to die down.

BUT

Watch carefully for signs of worsening.

Home Treatment: Bronchitis

- **Is he a nice pink colour**, still smiling at you and drinking his bottles? Then the bronchiolitis is very likely mild and can be treated at home.

- **Give lots of liquids** as he may have a temperature.

- **If feeding is difficult**, try breastfeeding or bottles, 'little and often'.

- **Lower any temperature** with ibuprofen or paracetamol.

- **If your child is coughing a lot**, prop him up a little with a rolled blanket under the mattress. Don't give cough medicine – sips of water are just as effective and much safer. Steam and menthol will not help.

- **Antibiotics** do not help; and they won't prevent it getting worse.

- **Keep washing your hands** as your child is infectious (disinfectant sprays are of no value as the virus is airborne).

- **Keep him away from day care** until he's back to his normal self.

- **It is normal to feel worse on Day Two,** when the infection peaks, then dies down.

- **Watch carefully for signs of worsening.** If it is still Day One and he is getting worse, contact your doctor. If there are serious breathing problems or he is feeding badly, get emergency help.

- **If it's severe**, he will be admitted to hospital. He may need oxygen and (if he is not feeding) intravenous fluids.

- **Apart from oxygen** for severe cases, nothing will ease his breathing until the virus works itself out. So I don't advise steroids, asthma inhalers, antiviral treatments or chest physiotherapy.

- **Don't change his milk feeding routines** as milk has not been proved to cause excessive mucus.

When bronchiolitis gets bad, it can be a little hard to distinguish from pneumonia.

Is It Pneumonia?

Pneumonia, which is a bacterial infection, strikes fear into parents. Signs that an infection may have moved down into his chest include:

- Fast breathing (remember that younger children have a higher breathing rate).

- A temperature of over 38.5°C.

- 🩹 Constant coughing.
- 🩹 The ribcage pulled in sharply and maybe grunting sounds when he breathes.
- 🩹 Sometimes there are chest pains.
- 🩹 Nostrils that are flared open to let in more air.
- 🩹 Lips and tongue have turned blue or purple because of lack of oxygen.
- 🩹 If the pneumonia is severe, your child will be quite limp (not eating or drinking) and will not notice what is going on around him.

He may have some (but not all) of these symptoms. Fast breathing is the one symptom that is a certainty – if your child is **not** breathing quickly then it is probably not pneumonia.

If he is pre-school age, the bacterium *Streptococcus pneumoniae* is the most likely cause of pneumonia. If he is school-going, it is more likely to be an atypical bacterium, *Mycoplasma pneumoniae*. This one is often called 'walking pneumonia' as he may seem quite well but a chest X-ray will show quite dramatic changes.

Home Treatment: Pneumonia

- ➕ **Call your doctor.** If pneumonia is severe, your child will be treated in hospital. More often, it will be mild and he will be treated at home under the care of your doctor.
- ➕ **Antibiotics** will be needed.
- ➕ **He will need plenty of fluids** and paracetamol because of the temperature.
- ➕ **Other treatments** such as steam, back clapping and herbal remedies will not solve the problem.

Children usually recover completely from pneumonia, without any after effects. He should not need a follow-up X-ray if he is back to full health and if the pneumonia was uncomplicated. The new pneumococcal vaccine is proving very successful in countries where it is available.

Is It Croup?

Adults get laryngitis – children get croup. It is very frightening (you will always remember the first time), and it is often worse in the lonely hours of night. Most croup is mild and a brief episode, but it can worsen. You are unlikely to miss the signs:

- 🩹 He has a very distinctive barking cough (like a seal).

- There's a 'hee' sound as he breathes in, known as 'stridor'.
- There is usually a low temperature.

Croup (laryngotracheobronchitis) is not a chest infection. It is caused by a parainfluenza virus, which makes the walls of his windpipe temporarily swell so it narrows. All that noise is from his efforts to breathe in more air. Young children are most affected because their windpipes are small and soft, which is why croup gets less common as they get older.

Or could it be whooping cough? If you are unsure, then it is probably not. The coughing spasms of whooping cough are quite frightening and the whoops are very definite.

Home Treatment: Croup

- **Steam** was the traditional solution for croup. A short stay in the bathroom with the hot taps pouring was believed to open the airways (it certainly calmed everyone down!). Closer examination, sadly, has found that it has no effect on the airways and it is not medically recommended any more. The hospital steam-tent is now a thing of the past.
- **Prop your child up** in bed with a pile of pillows. If he is a baby, prop him with a rolled blanket under the mattress.

HOW TO PROP UP A COT MATTRESS

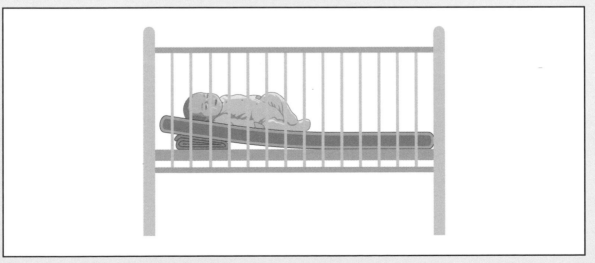

- **Stay with your child** and reassure him until the breathing eases.
- **Antibiotics** are not needed.
- **He can go to the crèche or playschool** if breathing has returned to normal and he is not too tired. It is usually a night affair that clears by morning.

- ✚ **Call your doctor** if you are concerned or the 'hee' sound gets worse. Either an oral steroid or a nebuliser with a steroid will be given.
- ✚ **Get emergency help** if your child is finding it hard to breathe or drink and his colour changes.

Is It Whooping Cough?

Whooping cough (pertussis) is now rare but we still see cases of it, in spite of vaccination. It is quite a dramatic illness, very upsetting to see and one to watch very carefully. These are the signs:

- ✚ He had a 'normal cold' for a week or two. Then the classic symptoms started.
- ✚ There are fits of uncontrollable coughing and a red face.
- ✚ Each fit is followed by a whooping sound (trying to get air) and vomiting.
- ✚ He usually has a slight temperature.
- ✚ He seems well (but weak) between spasms.
- ✚ The coughing spasms can go on for at least six weeks, and then they start to fade.

It's very infectious, but mostly **before** the coughing starts. It stays infectious until the antibiotics take hold. The condition is caused by *Bordatella pertussis*. Your doctor may diagnose it or send a nasal swab for laboratory testing.

Home Treatment: Whooping Cough

Whooping cough is a long, hard struggle and it may take up to three months to shake it off – you need to contact your doctor. It is prevented by vaccination.

Or Something Else?

- ✚ A foreign body breathed into lungs, a speciality of toddlers; tiny pieces of Lego and peanuts are the usual offenders.
- ✚ If he gets chesty symptoms regularly (with a wheeze) he may have asthma.
- ✚ Tuberculosis is still a problem in Western Europe. But if your child had a BCG vaccination, he should be immune or, at worst, get a mild version. He will have a chronic cough, have night sweats with a temperature, lose weight and usually (but not always) be quite sick.

➕ Cystic fibrosis and problems with the immune system are rare. But if his 'chest problems' are not going away and he is not gaining weight, your doctor may need to look at the possibility.

The Inside Track

Every time a child breathes in, air enters the body and travels down the breathing passages (respiratory tracts). We talk about them in three parts: the nose and throat (upper tract); the windpipe (middle tract, which you can feel at the front of the neck); and the chest and lungs (lower tract). The lungs are a collection of branch-like passages (bronchi and bronchioli) that end up in tiny sacs called alveoli. These have the important job of releasing oxygen into the bloodstream and taking carbon dioxide out.

Generally speaking, sniffs and sneezes mean an infection in the upper respiratory tract. Coughs and wheezes mean infection in the lower tract. When children cough or sneeze, they are vacuuming their airways and expelling extra mucus. This is usually a signal that their immune system is fighting something – a virus, bacteria – that has infected the airways. The lymph nodes (the glands) produce antibodies to kill the germs and give immunity from them in future. The glands swell while they are producing (feel the sides of the neck and you may notice it) and the swelling fades as soon as the germs are finished off.

OUR BREATHING SYSTEM

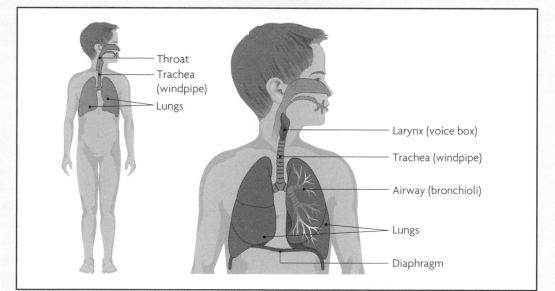

- Throat
- Trachea (windpipe)
- Lungs
- Larynx (voice box)
- Trachea (windpipe)
- Airway (bronchioli)
- Lungs
- Diaphragm

Are chest X-rays useful? They can be disappointing because they often cannot tell you what has caused the infection – whether a virus or bacteria. So we usually limit them to children with serious breathing problems.

Always remember that chest and breathing infections are easily spread through droplets. Keep out of the line of fire and keep hands washed.

Q&A

Q **My child seems to be prone to chest infections. Should we try giving him immunostimulants to prevent them?**

A Immunostimulants are a recent class of drugs and they were developed to fight infection by prevention. They work by stimulating the natural immune responses in the body and are now used to prevent serious respiratory infections.

Trials have shown that they can reduce – quite considerably – the number of infections in children who are susceptible. But we need to be a little cautious, because so far there have been no large controlled trials and (though they are approved for safe use) the effects of the drugs are not fully clear. I would be slow to use them.

Q **Ever since he started school this year, he has been snuffling. Should I give him vitamin tablets or something like echinacea?**

A The classic image of 'snot-nosed' schoolchildren came from somewhere. On average they get between six and eight viral infections a year (the immune system has a crash course but toughens up after a year or two) and most will heal by themselves.

If he is snuffling a lot, but seems to be well otherwise, I would simply let nature take its course. It is very likely to be an upper respiratory infection and he will settle down.

There really is no reliable evidence that vitamin tablets and herbal remedies will **stop** him getting colds. Echinacea has become popular and research supporting it is promoted in the media but we are still waiting for a medical breakthrough and it has been linked to rashes in children. As for vitamin C, the benefits are still unclear. We know from 30 trials involving 11,350 people that taking vitamin C does not prevent colds. If it is taken before the symptoms start, it may simply shorten a cold. Of course, vitamins in the child's diet will serve the same purpose. Taking 200 milligrams or more of vitamin C a day – once a cold starts – has little effect. Remember that it is possible to over-dose on vitamins and minerals. If your child is healthy and eats a varied diet, he should not take multivitamins. He will be at greater risk of vitamin overdose, which can be dangerous.

Far more useful for your child would be daily fresh air and exercise – especially in winter when he is liable to be sealed in for long periods with every prevalent virus. If somebody smokes in your house, he will get more colds and chest infections. And forget cough bottles. They are a massive national expense, for precious little gain.

Q He gets frequent sore throats – should I do more for them?

A Most sore throats are caused by a virus and if your child gets one he should recover naturally within a week – without any treatment. They rarely develop into anything more complicated. It is quite normal for the sore throat to get worse for a few days and then improve.

With a sore throat, he will find swallowing painful and may also have a cough, temperature or headache. You may feel swollen glands in his neck. The best advice is to give him plenty of fluids and give him paracetamol or ibuprofen at regular intervals while the throat is sore (not just when needed). Gargling can soothe his throat a little. Antibiotics will not be needed unless it is not easing after a few days.

Sore throats are quite common and your child should grow out of them. But if he is missing school frequently because of a very sore throat with a high temperature (or has enlarged tonsils) I would consider a tonsillectomy.

Baby Chest Infections

🐻 Your baby is very likely to get bronchiolitis at least once – and probably more often.

🐻 Always talk to your doctor if your baby has any breathing problems, especially if these date from birth. If you breastfed for the first few months, your child will fight infections better.

🐻 'Wheezy babies' are very common. It may simply be the after-effects of an infection but sometimes it can be a forerunner to asthma. Or your baby is a passive smoker.

Red Alert

CALL THE DOCTOR IF YOU ARE WORRIED. YOU CAN HELP BY ASSESSING HIM FIRST AT HOME:

✚ Count the breathing rate over a minute (it varies with age but over 40 breaths a minute needs help).

✚ Is the chest heaving in and out, with diaphragm and muscles working hard?

✚ Has the skin turned bluish around the lips or tongue?

✚ Is the child making a grunting sound?

✚ Does the child have a high temperature?

GET EMERGENCY HELP IF:

✚ Your child is under three months, breathing quickly and coughing. Especially if his lips are blue and he sometimes seems to stop breathing.

✚ He is having serious difficulty breathing.

✚ His chest draws in sharply with every breath.

SCENARIO 3 The seven-year-old schoolgirl has had an unfortunate accident in school. Her underpants are slightly soiled and she and her parents are mortified and terrified it might happen again. It is very tough for her and a negative reaction at home will really shatter her (already fragile) confidence.

Scenario 2 and **3 only** are constipated.

THE BRISTOL STOOL CHART

Type 1		Separate hard lumps, like nuts (hard to pass).	
Type 2		Sausage-shaped but lumpy.	
Type 3		Like a sausage but with cracks on its surface.	Healthy stool
Type 4		Like a sausage or snake, smooth and soft.	Healthy stool
Type 5		Soft blobs with clear-cut edges (passed easily).	
Type 6		Fluffy pieces with ragged edges, a mushy stool.	
Type 7		Watery, no solid pieces. Entirely liquid.	

The Bristol Stool Chart was developed in 1997 to help doctors to distinguish different forms of human faeces. Where is your child's stool on the chart?

Is It Constipation?

It can be hard to know if your child is constipated. Parents often insist that there are no signs, and misread an exaggerated attempt to perform. 'She goes several times a day. It's soft, so how could it be constipation?' But they may also agree that small amounts of liquid are staining her clothes.

Officially, constipation is 'the infrequent passage of hard stools, causing distress to a child'.

⊕   Look out for small stool 'pellets' when she is on the toilet. These are one of the most frequent signs of constipation.

- Or the opposite – large stools like tree trunks.
- Is she starting to jiggle about, is she grimacing?
- If her underpants soil, it is a definite.
- Use the Bristol Stool Chart (above) to decribe her stool.

Or Something Else?

Could it be serious? Yes, but it's rare. Less than 5 per cent of constipated children have a medical issue, such as Down syndrome, hypothyroidism or cystic fibrosis. Usually, they will already be identified. They will test your child for Hirschsprung's disease if she: is seriously constipated, was slow to pass meconium (the first, black, bowel motion), isn't thriving and has a seriously swollen tummy. Children with Hirschsprung's disease have permanent constipation from birth. But, before you panic, it is exceptionally rare and affects fewer than 1 in 7,000 births.

Some parents worry that there could be a serious psychological problem. In fact, very few cases are referred because of this. But some children who soil can develop tremendous problems with confidence. A very tiny minority of children will have encopresis – they pass normal stools in abnormal places. These cases are best managed by a child psychiatrist.

Soiled Clothes

Some parents are puzzled when their constipated child suddenly shows all the signs of diarrhoea – by soiling her underpants. In fact, this is a severe case of constipation. 'Overflow soiling' happens when soft stools leak from behind a lump of hard stool in an over-stretched rectum.

If she stains her underpants, as a general rule she has constipation, not diarrhoea. Up to 5 per cent of young school children soil (boys are three times more likely than girls), and it's almost always because of severe constipation. It's often made worse by the reaction of everyone else: teasing, rejection or disgust. Or by parents who find it hard to hide their anger or helplessness. Some parents even think that their child is soiling deliberately and their negative reactions simply make everything worse.

When training junior doctors about constipation, I teach them to handle parent and child with great sensitivity. Try it yourself, especially with soiling. It is the most likely approach to succeed.

The Diet Myth

Parents usually assume that diet is the biggest concern with constipation. The reality is that, for children, toileting routines are the main problem.

Think of the frenetic lifestyles we, and our children, lead. There is no time these days to lie in a field and simply gaze at the sky. Children often don't take time to go to the toilet and the nasty effects build up. To some degree, constipation can be learned. Your child with a tendency learns to associate the toilet with pain. Then fears build up to the point where she avoids the school toilets.

This is insidious and not a lot to do with diet.

Regular toilet routines are a must if you want to solve constipation. Give her more time on the toilet. It really is a delicate art and needs a relaxed space in her life. Make sure she is comfortable with the person on Toilet Patrol — is it a hassled crèche assistant or teacher? Are you rushing the child every day from playschool to shops to bed? She is probably learning to hold it back.

Diet can make matters worse, or better. Surprisingly, there have been no clinical trials to prove that dietary change (increased fluids, fruit juices or dietary fibre) reduces constipation. However, some case-control studies have shown that constipated children eat less fibre and if a child is reared on fast food this will certainly aggravate any problem. But changes in diet are not likely to help if the prime cause of the constipation is 'holding back'. It makes sense to look at toilet routines and diet together.

Fibre for Kids

Foods to be recommended:

* Fibre-rich breakfast cereals (porridge oats, muesli, All Bran)
* Dried apricots, prunes and figs
* Baked and kidney beans
* Lentils
* Sweetcorn
* Brown bread
* Blackberries and raspberries
* Passion and kiwi fruit

Be choosy with bananas. A ripe banana can relieve constipation, but a green (high-starch) banana can actually cause it. Bran is an extra source of fibre, but it is not recommended for young children as it may affect absorption of zinc and iron. It's far better for your child to eat foods rich in fibre than to add bran to food.

How Often Should They Deliver?

Don't get hung up on stool quotas, but get to know your **own** child's bowel pattern. Studies have shown averages for different age groups, but the range of so-called 'normal' is actually very wide. It is not a courier service.

AVERAGE PATTERNS OF DAILY BOWEL MOTIONS

Age	Number of Bowel Motions
First few weeks	4
4 months old	2
4 years old	1

(But a healthy four-year-old can have anything from three a day to three a week! And a baby may not perform for two days.)

The Inside Track

It is not only nine-year old schoolboys – maybe we are all secretly fascinated by our bowels. For those who want a closer look at how constipation works, read on.

When stool enters your child's rectum, the rectum distends and contracts, making her want to empty her bowels. This is a natural urge and it causes an important muscle, the internal anal sphincter, to relax. Out comes the stool. If she wants to have a say in the matter, she has two powerful weapons – muscles known as the external anal sphincter and the levator ani. All she has to do is tighten these muscles and – great – the door stays firmly shut. What's more, the urge to deliver lessens.

After a while, water loss makes the stool hard and more difficult to pass, and now she has absolutely no intention of letting it out. This makes the lower colon increasingly swollen as the stool builds up. Surprisingly, perhaps, this reduces any sensation in her rectum and makes her urge to perform even more irregular.

But something has to give. When the rectum is very distended, softer stool starts to leak out around the lump of hard stool. Because of the lack of sensation, she will not notice it until she has soiled her clothes. Then we have severe constipation.

Home Treatment: Constipation

Most constipation problems can be sorted out at home. I always advise new toilet and diet routines – but keep them low-key (don't have a family council or toilet rules). Keep it up for at least six months if you want to retrain her.

Some parents go into overdrive, seeing every spare moment as a toilet opportunity and analysing every food for fibre content. There are far easier approaches.

- **Remove any blame** as the first, reassuring step. Nobody is at fault here, neither you nor your child.

- **Sit your child on the toilet for 10–15 minutes after each home meal.** Make it fun with storybooks, toys or favourite music. Praise her gently when she performs or stays soil-free. Her gastro-colic reflex is most active after breakfast and this is the most important time. A footstool is more comfortable and will keep her hips fully flexed. Sit her three times a day whether she has a bowel motion or not. It can work wonders, as long as you keep it up. (Grateful parents swear by it!)

- **Have a quiet talk with her schoolteacher** about toilet time in school.

Sitting your child on the potty after each meal can help with constipation

- **Look at her diet**:
  - Give lots of water or diluted fruit juice.
  - Avoid too much cow's milk. It can fill her and leave little room for other foods that have fibre.
  - Try safe, natural laxatives such as prunes, rhubarb or liquorice. Kiwi fruit is a great mover and shaker.
  - Dried apricots, baked beans and other fibre-rich foods will help. (See Fibre for Kids on page 42.) Don't fill her up on processed (low-fibre) foods.
- **Look for signs of an anal tear or blood streaks.** This could be caused by hard stools and would certainly be adding to her woes. It will heal naturally once everything softens again.
- **Use a stool softener for a while**, with medical advice. This will take some of the stress out of toileting and reduce her fears. Getting it into her may be a challenge, but it is relatively tasteless. Sneak it into her food until she starts flowing again. Don't be horrified if it takes several months until you taper off the dose.
- **Get your child moving.** Exercise will keep digested food moving through the intestines.
- **Abdominal massage therapy** seems to help constipated bowels to move (get some guidance in this).
- **Acupuncture won't help** chronic constipation.
- **If your child soils**, confirm that it is constipation with your doctor. She'll need laxatives and (more important) a new toileting routine.
- **Don't rush toilet training.** It's a voluntary action and your child has full control. Most delays in toileting happen because of fear of sitting on the toilet. You don't need conflict.
- **Biofeedback** trials in children have been disappointing.
- **Flax seeds and senna** are often used as natural remedies for constipation. They can be effective, but I don't advise them for children.

Most parents avoid laxatives, believing that they make for lazy bowels. There is no evidence to back this up and some can be useful if nothing is working. Macrogol is a stool softener that can be used safely and has a higher success rate (with fewer side effects) than lactulose. It passes through the gut without being absorbed. It draws water into the bowel and increases the water content of the stools, softening them. (She can actually take up to 12 sachets a day.) But bowel stimulants (such as bisacodyl or senna) are different – they propel stool towards the exit and, though they are safe, I don't advise using them for long periods.

If the child's routines don't change, the problem will resurface very quickly. I've found that the greatest barrier to a solution is when parents let slide the 15-minute 'toilet sit' after meals.

THE RIGHT SITTING SYSTEM

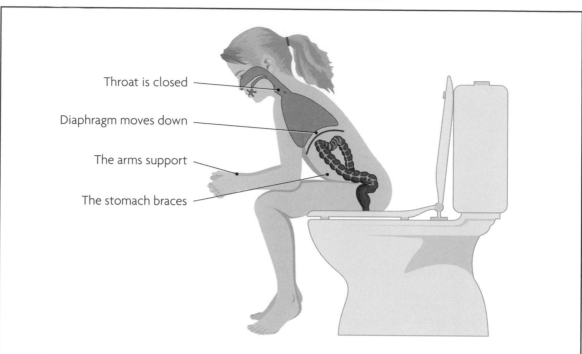

Throat is closed

Diaphragm moves down

The arms support

The stomach braces

The right way to open the bowels is shown here. Your child's position on the toilet is crucial and the best position is squatting – it lets the anal canal open fully. Make sure her feet are supported if she's small.

Q&A

Q The constipation has got so bad that, short of force, I can't even persuade her to go into the bathroom. Should I push it?

A No, not unless you want to prolong everything. You will need a lot of time to get it solved – be ready to drop everything for the first week. (Remember the agonies of toilet training?)

Try to break the association between the toilet room and fear of pain. If your child has dug in deep, you may need to be drastic about this and change the whole feel of the room. Fill it with teddies, throw in a beanbag, get a fun toilet seat or add a flashy mobile – whatever will surprise her. Have something special to hand such as a new music system, a musical box or a wind-up toy. At first, just cuddle up on the beanbag and read a story; later, try sitting her on the toilet lid while she listens, then eventually read to her on the open seat.

A stool softener may also help. When she finally does perform (and she will and will need lavish praise) it won't be such an ordeal. Don't rush it and, above all, don't force her to sit on the toilet. She holds all the cards here.

Q **My baby is nearly four months old and is breastfeeding. The problem is that her bowel movements seem to be very erratic. She might not have a motion for three days at a time. Why is she constipated?**

A In fact, she very likely is not constipated. She is still very young and everything will tend to be a little irregular until she settles down – and this includes the bowel motions. It is not unusual for a baby to delay a motion for two or three days. And it is also possible to have several motions a day – even more than the daily 'average' of two. I wouldn't be concerned so long as she is growing and is otherwise healthy. She will eventually settle into a regular routine.

Q **Surely some tests are needed to make sure it's only constipation?**

A Diagnosing constipation is relatively easy and few tests are normally needed. But sometimes an abdominal X-ray or ultrasound can be helpful to convince parents (and the patient) that this is indeed the problem. I would not rush into tests, however.

Q **She soils her underpants quite frequently and I'm not sure what to do about it.**

A Always remember that soiling means constipation and treat it accordingly. The secret to success in solving it is to be quite generous with stool softeners in the early stage (to ease things) and to have a 15-minute toilet sitting routine at least twice a day until the soiling has stopped and she realises again when she needs to go to the toilet. It could take several months to change her habits and stop the soiling completely.

Baby Constipation

A constipated baby is less common, but it happens. After all, your child is getting used to a lot of changes in her diet and some hiccups can be expected. Most come with a change of milk feeds, or when moving from the breast to formula milk. Baby is constipated when bowel motions are not frequent and cause her a lot of distress. You can do a lot to help:

- Try a different brand of formula milk (but don't keep changing milks).
- If your child is on solids, give more puréed vegetables and fruits.
- Give regular water between feeds.
- Talk to your doctor about stool softeners if she is very distressed.
- Don't reduce her milk – she needs it. Follow the standard guidelines.
- Don't change to soya milk. She will react in the same way.
- Avoid enemas and suppositories if possible.

Guide to Toilet Training

Toilet training is not something to rush, even when his playschool place depends on getting him out of nappies. Your child will become toilet trained when he is ready. Not when you or his grandparents or his playschool want. After all, it's a voluntary action and he is ultimately in control.

But you can help things along. Most children will be fully toilet trained by the time they are three years old (some much earlier), but when they achieve it depends hugely on the individual child. Boys tend to get there later than girls.

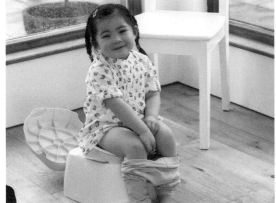

- Don't start too early, don't rush it and don't make it a fighting matter. Keep it as relaxed as you can.

- Eighteen months to two years of age is the earliest time to consider toilet training. By then, he will be able to follow basic instructions.

- Getting him to sit on a potty or toilet is the first step. Some parents find a training seat useful (a small seat that fits over your toilet seat). Don't use pull-up nappies, as they will slow things down.

- Look out for signs that he is about to perform. A slight change in posture, a change of expression or colour in his face. He may seem restless. Then lift him onto a potty or toilet seat and make it a game. If anything comes out, praise him. It will encourage a repeat. Success is most likely within 20 minutes of a meal, so stand by at these times.

- He needs to learn how to sit on the toilet or potty before learning to open his bowels on it. Start to sit him regularly on the toilet, but make it a relaxing event. Chat to him, read to him. Eventually the great day will come when he performs – and not because you caught him just in time. Lavish him with praise and ring or text all interested parties – of course it is over the top, but it works a treat.

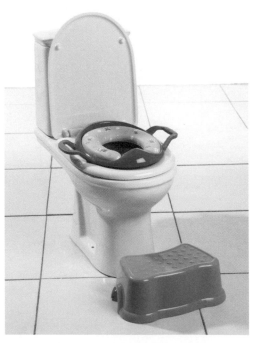

A training seat can be useful in encouraging your child to sit on the toilet

- Delays in toilet training do happen, most often because of fear of sitting on the toilet. Be patient and don't fight over it. A relaxed approach is the best policy.
- If he gets constipated, or if there is any kind of family crisis, put a hold on training until the problem has gone.
- Don't impose deadlines for toilet training – you are very likely to be disappointed. But do make time to work with him on it.

Above all, avoid conflict. He holds all the trump cards.

Red Alert

When you cannot break the cycle at home, it is quite sensible to visit your doctor. It'll usually be a two-stage solution: a 'stick of dynamite' approach (with medication) to clear the blockage; and toilet routines to avoid repeat problems.

In extreme cases, your child may need a short period in hospital. Some children resist other treatments and cannot seem to relax the external sphincter.

If your child is under three months old, has constipation and is not thriving, she must see a doctor.

Chapter 5
Eczema

'He had lovely skin, but now he gets this rash on his face and chest. It's all very dry and flaky and seems to itch a lot. He's started rolling around in his cot at night time and every chance he has he scratches at his skin. I've tried rubbing cream on, but it still looks a bit of a mess.'

The 'Yuck Factor'

The itching is probably the worst part. Your child lies there, scratching away as if his bed is infested. He is not sleeping (and neither are you) and for many this is the real headache with eczema.

Or maybe it is the look of it: his red, scabby skin that people cannot help staring at. Doctors see eczema simply as a skin disease, but for you and your child it is a disfigurement. Apart from the discomfort, he has to cope with the 'yuck factor', the squeamish reactions from other people – especially his pals. At least he's not alone:

- ⊕ One in five children has what we call atopic eczema.
- ⊕ Most will grow out of it before they start school.
- ⊕ It is rarely severe.
- ⊕ It's a skin barrier problem and keeping the skin moist is half the battle.

If it does linger beyond childhood, it'll be mainly in the joint areas (wrists and knees). Fewer than 5 per cent of children have really serious eczema where – unfortunately – over 20 per cent of their body is covered in the rash. Very important, eczema is **not infectious** and your child can't spread it to other children.

Is It Eczema?

It's usually easy enough to spot eczema. There are tell-tale signs:

- ⊕ The skin is dry and itchy.
- ⊕ There is often a family history of allergies.
- ⊕ The skin problem started early (under two years old).
- ⊕ The rash started on the face, then in front of the elbows or ankles and behind the knees.

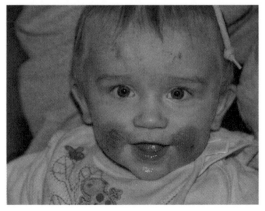

Eczema

These are the flashpoints, but the rash can turn up almost anywhere. It'll be dry and flaky, but get wet and gooey if it gets infected. The real nasty (a worst-case) scenario has it all – dry, red skin all over the body that really itches. In fact, if it does not itch, it is usually not eczema.

ECZEMA

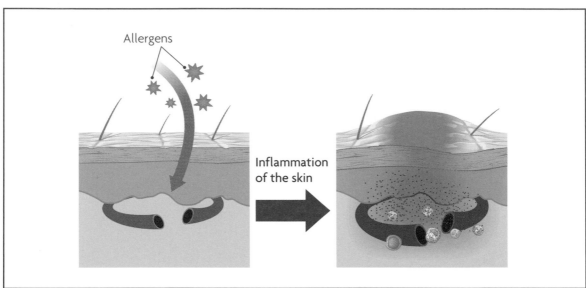

If your child has eczema, he will get skin infections more often and these really help the skin to flare up. It's a vicious circle.

Or Something Else?

A **FOOD ALLERGY** can show as an itchy, blotchy rash and sometimes you will see puffiness around the eyes. But it's less common than you think (for over 90 per cent of children with eczema, food allergies are not the cause). And the reaction will be sudden, usually within fifteen minutes of eating the food. There will be a dramatic rash flare-up or vomiting, wheezing, even tongue swelling.

If your child has small, itchy blisters – usually between the fingers, toes and on the soles of the feet – then it's more likely to be **SCABIES**, which your doctor can easily treat (see page 181).

With **IMPETIGO**, you will see a yellow, crusty rash and it will not itch very much (see page 164).

 Many babies get **SEBORRHOEIC DERMATITIS**. The skin is red and flaky (on the scalp this is known as 'cradle cap') but not too itchy. It usually clears up quickly but moisturising creams and baths will help.

PSORIASIS is much rarer in young children. You will see red, scaly patches on his skin, but it does not itch.

The Inside Track

Do food allergies account for the rise in eczema? No – it's a skin barrier flaw and he is very likely born with it. His eczema is more often triggered by what he touches or breathes than what he eats.

Think of eczema skin as a sensor. It is especially allergic and it can react to the slightest thing. The eczema will flare up easily and this has quite an impact on his quality of life.

A lot of it is genetic. It tends to run in families and often comes with a bunch of other allergies, such as asthma or hay fever. Experts now believe that there is an eczema gene – if your child has it, he is more likely to get eczema – but will identifying the gene make any difference? Possibly not. Triggers can make it worse. They don't actually cause the eczema, but they will spark off a rash if the skin is too dry. I am usually less worried about the triggers and more concerned about keeping the skin in good shape.

The skin is a physical barrier that protects the body and holds moisture within it. With eczema, this barrier becomes impaired so that it cannot hold enough moisture in the skin cells. The skin becomes dry and starts to crack, making it easier for allergens to enter.

How does this work? Some 80 per cent of the body's outer skin (the epidermal cells) is made of keratin protein. As the cells naturally rise towards the skin surface, the amount of keratin in them increases. By the time the cells reach the outer skin, they are dead and are normally made entirely of keratin. If there is a deficiency, the skin looks cracked and flaky as it sloughs off. Keratin needs water to make it pliable and when there is not enough water it crumbles and the cells can no longer stay together. The normal skin oils also get depleted and as a result some of the natural moisture escapes.

We need to find ways of trapping water. Moisturisers simply act on the body's natural oils and hold water longer.

Pimecrolimus will stop eczema flaring up, but I would use it with caution. Limit it to second-line treatment for eczema on the head and neck, where steroids do not work.

Home Treatment: Eczema

You can do a lot to prevent the eczema flaring up. And to ease it:

- **Your child will not need to be tested for allergies**, unless the eczema is severe.

- **Throw out** every soap and bubble bath on your shelves.

- **Use a soap substitute** from now on. Ask your chemist for a good emulsifying ointment or aqueous cream instead. Use it instead of shampoo if your child is under one year.

- **Lavish on the moisturiser** as often as you can and over the whole body, not just the affected area. Ideally, every few hours. (He can keep a tube at school.) Keep creaming him, even when the eczema is clear and while he is using other treatments. Use even more cream when the eczema flares up. Apply it in downward strokes (following the direction of hair growth) to avoid blocking his hair follicles.

- **Don't ban any foods.** They are almost certainly not the cause.

- **Ideally, bath every day.** Give a warm bath and always add moisturising oil (eczema-recommended) in the water. Rub moisturiser into the skin as soon as he gets out.

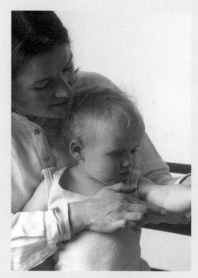

Applying moisturiser every few hours can help prevent eczema flaring up

- **Put antiseptic oils** in the bath too, if his skin flares up. A weekly antiseptic bath can also prevent it.

- **Always double rinse his clothes** (if you hand rinse you will see how much soap stays behind). Fabric conditioners are bad news. But (despite popular belief) non-biological washing powders are no better for eczema than biological ones. Wash all new clothes before he wears them.

- **Stick to cotton** (or polyester-cotton) clothes if you can. Cotton soothes and some fabrics irritate.

- **Change the bedclothes** frequently and use a mattress cover.

- **Keep the bedroom cool** at night as heat can set him off.

- **Catch itching quickly.** Use a sedating antihistamine and calamine-impregnated gauze. Baths will also help and you can try a baby sleepsuit or mitts to stop the scratching.

- **'Wet wraps'** can help if itching is bad and you want to stop him scratching away the cure. After you rub on the cream or steroid, wrap a bandage around the area a few times (like a mummy), until the outside is dry.

- **Keep his nails short;** consider bandaging his skin if you cannot keep those tiny nails away.

- In winter, **open windows or go outdoors** as heating and lack of ventilation will make his skin problems worse.

- **Treat any skin infection quickly.** Don't give the eczema something juicy to work on.

- There are many natural remedies, but **always check the list of ingredients**. Do they contain steroids and do they in fact cause irritation? Olive oil can be a natural alternative in the bath, but I would stick to moisturisers on the skin. The benefits of aloe vera for eczema is not clear and I'm slow to recommend it.

If it is not easing, have a word with your doctor.

- **He may need a topical steroid** rubbed into the skin (only the affected area) once a day but do keep moisturising him while he's taking the steroid! I prefer ointments to creams (the preservatives in these creams can irritate the skin). Keep moisturising him when using steroids, but leave an hour's space. Don't use strong steroids on the face or neck (they thin the skin).

- **If steroids don't work**, the doctor may prescribe tacrolimus (but not for babies) or pimecrolimus. It should not be used for mild eczema and is only a last resort for severe cases. Don't use it under bandages unless your dermatologist advises it. The antibiotic tetracycline is used with some skin conditions but not for children under twelve years.

- **Antibiotics with steroids** are generally not a good idea.

- **Phototherapy (ultraviolet light treatment)** has had some success for children with more severe eczema. But it needs medical supervision.

I would aim for short bursts of steroids and long 'holiday' intervals of simple moisturising. And the golden rule is: generous dollops of moisturising cream – but light fingertips of steroid cream.

BUT

Always check a rash with your doctor, if you are concerned or if your child seems off colour.

Q&A

Q If I change his diet, will it help?

A People would love to prove a link between eczema and food allergy, but it is just not stacking up. Eczema caused by food is actually quite rare. In fact, researchers have found that most children with eczema did not improve when foods were taken out of their diet. Even in severe cases, fewer than 10 per cent will improve when put on a food elimination diet (where one food is completely removed for a time) – a tiny group of children.

Often parents are so obsessed about diet that no one actually treats the child's skin. So nothing improves. Interestingly, researchers have shown that when these parents start to work on the skin, they worry less about food, and report fewer food reactions.

Skin care is much more important to your child than diet changes, unless there is a very clear link between the eczema and a specific food. If there is, stop that food for six weeks and see if the rash improves. In reality, it's more likely to affect an infant and it usually means excluding cow's milk (by switching his formula) or eggs from the diet, and always with medical advice. In addition, do keep moisturising.

If your child is under six months, is bottle-fed and has bad eczema, there is a small chance that he may be allergic to cow's milk. Your doctor will advise a trial change to a hypoallergenic formula for six weeks. But he will also need to see a dermatologist. Don't try goat's milk as it is not good for him at this age. And please do not exclude fruit from his diet, as citric acid does not cause his eczema.

Q I've been given steroid ointment and our doctor said to use it sparingly. How much should I use?

A A good guide to the amount to use is the Fingertip Measure. Squirt a piece like toothpaste along the top part of your child's index finger. This will be enough to treat an area of eczema the size of the two palms of your hand. If you follow this, a twice-daily application will be enough to control the eczema in most cases. It is important to use the least powerful steroid that works and to use it sparingly.

Q There's a confusing choice of moisturising creams in the shops. Which do I buy? Could he be allergic to any?

A The best cream is the one your child will use regularly. You're right – the choice is very wide, but any of these will work if they get lathered on every day: emulsifying ointments, aqueous cream, 50/50 liquid paraffin in soft white paraffin. Look for creams that are recommended for dry skin or eczema. Some people are puzzled that moisturising creams (emollients) are also used as soap substitutes. They are, and they work.

Q Could the eczema be caused by stress? My three-year-old started playschool recently and that's when it started.

A Stress is unlikely to be the cause with a small child. What's more likely is dry skin reacting to something external – his first woollen coat? An overheated room? He will certainly get stressed by the itching, so you need to start creaming his skin quickly.

Q His eczema was well controlled until recently, but now it has flared up and his skin is very red and moist. What should I do?

A Almost certainly, he has an infection on top of his eczema and this has caused the flare-up. He needs to see his doctor, who will prescribe oral antibiotics to settle it down. All that skin scratching probably led to the infection. But if the flare-up is dramatic, we have to consider herpes infection and he may need to see a dermatologist.

Baby Eczema

Eczema is mainly a baby thing. It usually starts before a child is two years old and then it flares up at intervals – especially when his skin is too dry. 'Cradle cap' normally dies away after the first few months.

Red Alert

If there are blisters, the skin is weeping or crusting or the eczema suddenly gets worse, it could be a skin infection. He may need antibiotics.

If the eczema is severe (covering over 20 per cent of the body and the skin is badly flaking or scaling), he may need to be seen by a specialist.

Eczema is never life threatening.

Chapter 6

Eye & Ear Problems

'She woke up hot and bothered and then started screaming and pulling at her ear. I've given her something for the pain but she's still crying. The same thing happened a few weeks ago but it seems worse this time.'

All that 'Gunge'

Eye and ear infections can be true pests in her early years, but they are seldom serious. Your child is still quite new to this world and her defences need time to mature.

- An earache that makes her cry is usually a middle ear infection.
- Red eyes are usually (but not always) caused by conjunctivitis.
- 'Glue ear' is invisible but can affect her hearing.
- Most eye and ear infections will heal naturally. Antibiotics are **not** always needed.

BUT

If she's a baby, or is very distressed (or if there are other, worrying symptoms), call her doctor.

Is It an Eye Problem?

CONJUNCTIVITIS A red eye usually means conjunctivitis – but not always. It is the most likely eye problem she will have. The signs are:

- Red and weeping eyes.
- The eyeball and inside eyelids are red and you see tiny blood vessels.
- On waking in the morning the eye is almost glued shut.

Conjunctivitis means that the lining of her eyelids and the surface of her eyeball (conjunctiva) are inflamed. It is usually for one of two reasons – an infection or an allergy. But always make sure there is no foreign body or chemical in the eye.

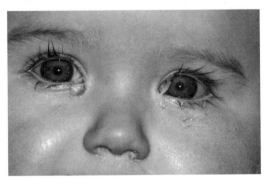

Conjunctivitis

Like a cold, the infection will usually sort itself out. Knowing what caused it can rule out antibiotics. Is it a virus? A bacterial infection? An allergy? The main clue is what is coming out of her eye. It is usually:

- A **virus** or an **allergy**, if the eye is watery and you see tiny amounts of stringy mucus when you pull her lower lid down. Her eye feels gritty. If both eyes are affected and are **itchy** too, it is usually an allergy (especially if she has a history of allergies).
- **Bacterial**, when there is thick, yellowish pus all around her eyelids and the corners of her eyes, and it keeps coming. When you wipe the lids, more appears.

STYE If there is only a small swelling on the eyelid, full of pus, it is probably a stye. A hair follicle will be inflamed but it will usually heal by itself. You can speed things up with hot compresses of cotton wool and water.

BUT

It's important to rule out a more serious eye problem (see Red Alert, page 172).

SQUINT Your child may seem to squint as a small baby, but this is not a worry. Under six months, her eyes don't move together in full 'binocular vision'. A squint after six months (or a 'lazy' eye or one that turns a little) is a different matter. It may only be an optical illusion (a wide nose or skin folds on the inside of her eye) but it needs to be reported. Squints are very common and tend to run in families; it is a muscle problem. The different muscles controlling eye movement do not pull as they should – so her two eyes do not look in the same direction.

The Inside Track: Eyes

When she sees, light enters her eye through her 'window', the cornea, which is the clear outer skin in front. It passes through her pupil and the light rays focus on the retina at the back of her eye. All the information about this light then travels from the retina to her brain and the pictures are interpreted.

INSIDE OUR EYE

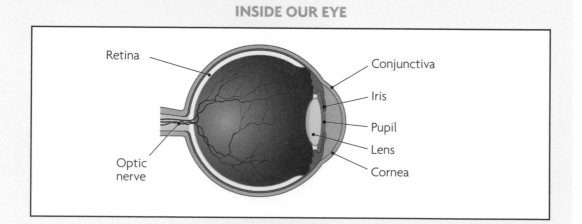

Her eyes have great powers of self-preservation – up to a point. Her eyelids will shut at the slightest irritation while her tears constantly wash her eyes and help to kill infections. And her nose, cheeks and forehead give her eyes some defence against blows. But although the eyeball is tougher than it seems, the outer eyes are the most vulnerable and that is where most injuries tend to happen.

Every movement of the eyes (up, down or sideways) is controlled by six muscles in the eyeball. To see correctly, both eyes have to move at the same time, the same distance and in the same direction. This is a difficult operation: our brain has to instruct one set of muscles to pull and the opposite set to relax. If the eye muscles are not co-ordinated, we get problems such as double vision.

Vision Milestones

If your child is not meeting the vision milestones below, talk to your doctor or optician. Until age three, any vision testing will need to be done by a trained person. You can informally check distance vision after that with pictures. Hopefully, your child will follow the vision milestones.

From week 1
She will turn towards a torch light.

By 2 months
She will follow your face if it moves and will smile back at you. Her eyes will move in the same direction. She will blink if startled.

By 3 months
She begins to discover her own body and will watch her hands moving. Her focus will also widen to action around her.

By 6 months
She will look around with interest and reach out for small objects. She'll fix on objects up to 30 centimetres away. Look out for any sign of a squint – after six months it is not normal.

By 9 months
She'll see and prod objects as small as crumbs.

By 12 months
She will point to anything you ask and grasp anything you hand her. She will recognise you from across the room and watch the world around her with great concentration.

Home Treatment: Eye Problems

Eye Infection (Conjunctivitis)

It will usually self-heal with a little home care, but watch for signs of worsening.

- **Foreign body.** First make sure there is nothing in the eye.

- **Keep the eyes clean.** Wipe each eye several times a day with boiled, cooled water (a tiny pinch of salt does seem to make a difference). Wipe from the nose to the outer edge of the eye and use different cotton balls for each eye. It is better than any antibiotic ointment.

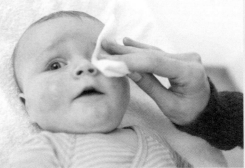

Use boiled, cooled water to clean an eye infection several times a day

- **Soothe the eye** with a cold, moist cloth. A herbal tea poultice will have the same effect. If it really itches, it is an allergy and you can try antihistamines or anti-inflammatory drops.

- **Colloidal silver drops** (a complementary health remedy) are **not** advised these days. There can be serious side effects, including skin discolouring.

- **Antibiotic ointments** in the eye will only help if it is a bacterial infection – and even then will only speed recovery a little. Don't jump in.

- **Wait for a day or two** and if there is no improvement get an ointment from your chemist. Ointments are better for children than drops as they stay longer on the eyelids and the child will wriggle less.

- **She's very infectious**, so keep everything separate until her eyes stop weeping – her own towel, facecloth, mug, cutlery – and wash your hands after touching her face (unless it's an allergy, in which case she is not infectious at all).

- **Can she return to school?** She can be infectious as long as her eyes are weeping, but it may not be realistic to wait so long. The school may insist that she uses an antibiotic ointment before she returns.

- **She should improve** after one to two days. Recovery may be slower if she has a cold or if it's an allergy. It may even get worse for a few days.

- **If it is an allergy**, try to avoid the soap, cream or whatever seems to cause it.

If she develops any of the Red Alert symptoms on page 72, see your doctor.

Squint

There are four ways of treating squints:

- **Patching** the good eye will make the squinting eye work harder.
- **Glasses** may be all that is needed.
- **Eye exercises** can help.
- **Surgery** can correct a squint, but it's usually for cosmetic reasons.

Is It an Ear Problem?

MIDDLE EAR INFECTION (otitis media) is the most likely ear infection. The chances of it increase if she goes to a crèche or if you smoke. There is a collection of symptoms:

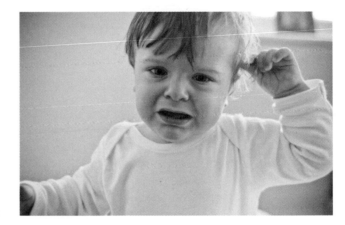

- Bad earache.
- Pulling or poking at her ear.
- A temperature.
- Being cranky, whining or even screaming.
- Off her food.
- Loss of hearing.
- Not sleeping.
- Thick, yellow pus that oozes from her ear.

Not every child will tick these boxes. A toddler or older child may scream with the pain. But the younger your child, the less likely she is to feel sore – a temperature is more likely. A look at her eardrum will confirm an infection. Most of the time, nature will sort it out for you, but if it worsens and she's very distressed, she'll need a doctor.

Look out for an ear oozing yellow pus. It usually means that her eardrum has burst to release trapped middle ear fluid – especially if the pain eases off. This is not quite as bad as it sounds and usually heals itself after a week. But it **must** be checked out.

AN OUTER EAR INFECTION is less likely. It often comes from a scratch, swimming in grubby water or a foreign body. The main difference is that it will itch and when you press on her ear, it'll hurt. The outside of her ear will be quite messy with yellow or crusty pus.

WAX There will always be a little wax in her outer ear – it is part of her natural ear hygiene. It is dark brown, very 'waxy' and harmless. It is only a problem if she develops a large plug of it and her hearing drops. But it is easily removed.

GLUE EAR You will not, in fact, see anything. But you may notice that she is not hearing as well as usual.

- Is she turning up the TV?
- Is she distracted at school?
- Does she hear you when you call gently?

If she had any ear infections recently, it could be glue ear.

This is simply the after-effects of an ear infection. Her middle ear will be full of excess fluid (thick and sticky, like glue), but now perfectly sterile. Draining it away is slow work. While the fluid is trapped, the eardrum cannot move efficiently – and sound waves become blocked. She may have lost up to 30 per cent of her hearing and this could also delay her speech.

It is seasonal and is worst during the colder months. In most cases, her ear will right itself without help, but it can take up to three months. It can be a real problem for children with medical conditions such as cleft palate, Down syndrome and chronic sinusitis.

HEARING LOSS usually means middle ear infections. One week she has a chest infection and everything gets blocked up (including hearing), then all is well again for a few months. Sometimes it can simply be a build-up of wax. More rarely, it can be nerve deafness.

Keep a good eye on your child's hearing if she has regular ear infections or if there is deafness in the family. It may slow her speech development. (If she was a premature baby or has had meningitis, there is a higher risk of deafness.) Trust your instincts if you think she's not hearing everything.

The Inside Track: Ears

To hear properly, any sound must reach the eardrum and set it vibrating. The sound then travels through the small bones of the middle ear to the inner ear where it becomes electrical signals that eventually reach the brain.

Most ear problems come from faulty drainage. There is always some fluid in the middle ear and more is produced when a virus or bacteria invade the area and it becomes inflamed. Usually, the excess fluid drains away down the Eustachian tube, which connects the middle ear to the throat.

INSIDE OUR EAR

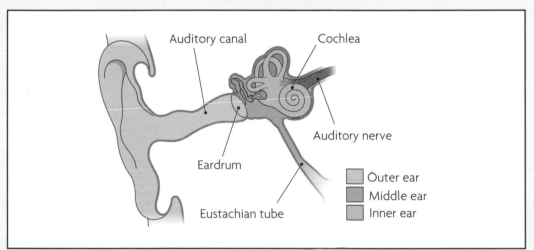

But if the tube gets blocked, the air in the middle ear creates a vacuum that draws fluid in from the ear lining. At first, this fluid is thin and watery but it eventually becomes thick and 'gluey'. As the fluid increases, it starts to affect hearing (because the eardrum and middle ear bones can't move freely) and pressure can cause painful earache. Children are more likely to get ear infections, partly because their immune system is still not as capable of fighting off infection. But it is also because their Eustachian tube is narrow and gets blocked easily. It is also shorter and cold germs have an easier journey from the throat.

Home Treatment: Ear Problems

Ear Infection

Very likely it will clear up by itself. You can usually 'wait and see' for a few hours, but err on the side of caution. If she's a baby or is very distressed, always talk to a doctor.

- **Give pain relief.** Paracetamol or ibuprofen will help. You can also get anaesthetic drops from the chemist.
- **Soothe the ear** with gentle heat. Try a warm, damp facecloth or a wrapped hot water bottle.
- **Antibiotics are not automatic.** If your child is less than one year old or is very unhappy, it's better to get antibiotics 'just in case'. But if she is older and coping, wait a little. Things should improve after a few hours.
- **Antihistamines, decongestants and steroids** will have no effect and should not be prescribed.
- **Swimming and full baths** are not a good idea until the infection has gone.
- **Fluid may stay in the ear** for a few weeks after the infection and affect hearing. Check her hearing after a few months if the ear infection was severe or if there have been repeat infections.
- **A daily antibiotic** may be prescribed for a short time, if the child has had at least three ear infections in the past three months. It will keep the ears germ-free.
- **Soothers (dummies)** should be used in small doses. They have been linked to ear infections.

Glue Ear

Most glue ear sorts itself out. But her ears and hearing should be checked every few months.

- **Watch her hearing** and make allowances for it.
- **Feed her upright** if she is a baby. The ears will not drain as easily lying down.
- **Don't smoke nearby.**
- **Relieve any pain** with paracetamol or ibuprofen.
- **Forget** antihistamines, decongestants or medicine that 'thins mucus' — they will make no difference.
- **Antibiotics** are not advised.
- **Oral steroids are not a good idea.** They only speed up the natural healing, they work for one-third of children and the price (the side effects of steroids) is too high.

➕ **Grommets**, surgically inserted in her ears, will drain away fluid but they are not for everyone. If she gets regular ear infections and it's affecting her hearing or speech, I would consider them. VEGF inhibitors are a new, but relatively untried, approach.

Wax

A little wax is quite normal, but a 'plug' of wax is a problem.

➕ **Melt it** with regular drops of warmed olive oil. Warm the oil in a teaspoon in the palm of your hand and drop it in gently. But don't poke at it with anything – it'll push it further in

➕ **If it's not shifting**, your doctor will prescribe drops or syringe her ear.

➕ **'Ear candling'** can cause serious damage and should not be used on children.

➕ **It is not a good idea to try syringing her ear yourself** – leave that to your doctor.

Baby Eyes and Ears

🐻 Babies are the biggest victims of eye and ear infections. Look out for conjunctivitis. Until she's a few months old, her tear ducts will be very immature and tears (the natural cleansers) may not flow readily. You can usually treat it at home by wiping her eyes in the normal way.

🐻 And watch for signs of an ear infection, especially a temperature – she'll need to see a doctor. Most of her ear infections will happen before she's two years old. Then, as her Eustachian tube gets bigger and more efficient, they'll start to peter out. But it's now known that a child whose parents smoke (or who's addicted to her dummy) is at a higher risk.

🐻 If you have breastfed her for at least three months, she will have fewer ear infections.

🐻 If your baby has a serious hearing defect, it is most likely to be picked up at birth. Many EU countries now have universal hearing screening.

If the twitching is more extreme and makes her eyelids close completely, it could be an eye infection. If it is conjunctivitis, her eyes will feel irritated or uncomfortable. Have a word with your doctor, if you have any doubts.

Q **She tends to get very painful ears when she flies. How can I help her on our next air trip?**

A Changes in atmospheric pressure can be very painful if her Eustachian tube is not working as it should. With barotraumas (there is a name for it!), she will have fluid behind her eardrum and flying will put extra pressure on her ears, causing pain and often loss of hearing. But it will usually resolve itself, though it can take a week or two. You can help to reduce it by feeding her (if she is a baby), giving her a sweet to suck or encouraging her to yawn – especially during take-off and landing. A decongestant before she flies can be useful too. But if she has an ear infection (otitis media), she really should not fly because there is always the risk of a burst eardrum.

Red Alert

CONTACT YOUR DOCTOR IF:

- She is a baby (or is very unwell) and you suspect an ear infection.
- Her ear oozes yellow pus and this eases any pain (it is probably a burst eardrum).
- Her eyes are badly affected. Is the whole eyeball red, but not her inner eyelids? Are the eyes so gritty and irritated that she can't keep them open?
- Her eyelids become very swollen (it may be a blocked tear duct).
- The mucus from her eye is bloodstained, yellow and creamy thick (it could be another infectious disease).
- If her eyes or ears don't improve within 24 hours.
- If she has regular infections, she may be referred to a specialist.

Chapter 7

Feeding Problems

'He's barely six weeks old and he vomits up after every bottle feed. My clothes are permanently a mess. What worries me even more, though, is his weight because he seems very light for his age.'

In General

I get regular calls about feeding problems – often from new parents. The usual worries are under-feeding, over-feeding, reflux or possible allergies; or a child who simply will not eat.

Feeding problems usually get sorted out with a little help and fewer than 5 per cent of them are serious.

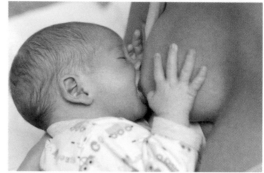

- Reflux is common in babies but rarely needs to be treated.
- Breastfeeding (if it works) is best for baby. But it is not instinctive and needs to be guided.
- Iron deficiency is a very real problem with children under two years.

As for food battles, remember that your child will always have the final say. He can clench his teeth.

Growth – The Yardstick

You should not worry unduly so long as he is growing and putting on weight. Babies always lose a little weight in their first week or two of life but after that, they should gain weight. This formula is a useful guide:

First 3 months	He returns to his birth weight by two weeks old and gains 200 grams a week after that
3–6 months	He gains 150 grams a week
6–9 months	He gains 100 grams a week
9–12 months	He gains 75 grams a week

It is also reassuring to track his growth on the **growth charts** (see pages 139–144).

Is It a Feeding Problem?

GASTRO-OESOPHAGEAL REFLUX always seems worse than it is.

- He brings up his bottle after every feed.
- He may be cranky.

Up to 50 per cent of babies have simple reflux and despite all the vomiting, they still thrive (the amount of vomiting is not usually as much as you think). If it is reflux, he is likely to grow out of it before his first birthday. And it will do him no harm. Your doctor can usually diagnose it by looking at the history of the problem, so barium X-rays or other tests are not necessary.

It is a weak muscle in the oesophagus that makes milk and acid come back up and it will bother him until the muscle toughens. But he will not starve. Very rarely, it can cause complications such as poor weight gain, irritability (if the oesophagus gets inflamed) or recurrent chest infections (if milk gets into the lungs).

Babies often **posset** and this can be mistaken for reflux – he'll splash back milk after most feeds. Maybe he gulped down too quickly or, like all babies, he is a self-regulating feeder and once he is full he simply spewed out the extras.

Home Treatment: Reflux

Reflux will sort itself out, as his muscles strengthen, but you can help.

- **The lying position** can ease things, but be careful. The best position is lying on his back with his head tilted up to 30° (put a blanket under the mattress). Sitting him in his carrycot or car seat will actually increase reflux.
- **Holding him upright** while feeding may help.
- **'Thickened feed' milks** cut down the amount of vomiting and this does relieve anxiety for parents.
- **Special formula milks** seem to help reflux and are worth trying after getting medical advice.
- **Some parents try chiropractic and baby massage**, but there is no evidence to show that it works.
- **Medication** is really not needed as most reflux is simple and rights itself with time. (But you will find several medications on the market that reduce acid production – some have still to prove their uses and some have side effects.)

Talk to your doctor if it is still a worry.

ABNORMAL NAPPIES He may have a few startling nappies, but don't worry. As your child grows and his feeds change, what comes out will change too.

Anything minor is very normal:

- 🧰 The first few days of life, he will pass meconium. This is green/black, sticky and pretty unpleasant.

- 🧰 If he is breastfed, he will move on to normal, loose stool that is orange-yellow. Enjoy the sweet smell as that will all change later (when he starts solids). It will tend to come out in little explosions and he will have up to eight motions a day.

- 🧰 If he is on formula milk, it will be quite different. Don't get a shock when you move him off the breast. He can have up to eight motions a day – or only one (much firmer) motion every second day.

Look out for:

Constipation In the first month or two he may seem to push it all out with a bit of effort and it is not constipation (unless he is very distressed). As he gets older, the signs will be clearer – small stool pellets or large stools like tree trunks and sometimes soiling of his clothes.

Diarrhoea If he is vomiting as well, it is more likely to be gastroenteritis. If he has a serious nappy rash with diarrhoea, it might be lactose intolerance. If your child is a toddler, you may see the odd undigested carrot or bean in the diarrhoea. This is fine and usually just means that everything has moved too quickly through his bowel.

Poor weight gain Does he seem too thin? The best yardstick is the average weight for his age (see the growth charts on pages 139–144). If you think your child is underweight, talk to your doctor, who will want to know:

- 🧰 Is he taking enough milk or solids?

- 🧰 Is there abnormal vomiting or diarrhoea?

- 🧰 Are there signs of an infection?

- 🧰 Is he developing normally, apart from his weight?

If nothing else seems to be wrong, he is probably not getting enough food.

Home Treatment: Abnormal Nappies

Abnormal nappies are not unusual. If he recently moved to formula milk, solids or has changed his formula milk, his nappies will look different too. But:

- **If the nappies are liquid**, try cutting down fruit juice.
- **Constipation** is not usually a problem with babies. But it can be helped with more fluids and a little brown sugar.
- **Rule out** gastroenteritis (see page 122) or lactose intolerance (page 80).

REFUSING TO EAT Lots of children simply will not eat. If your child is growing and full of energy, I would not worry too much. He will not starve and his eating habits should improve with age and with a little help. It is stressful, but I would only be concerned if:

- His weight is low for his age.
- There are signs of stress during feeding.

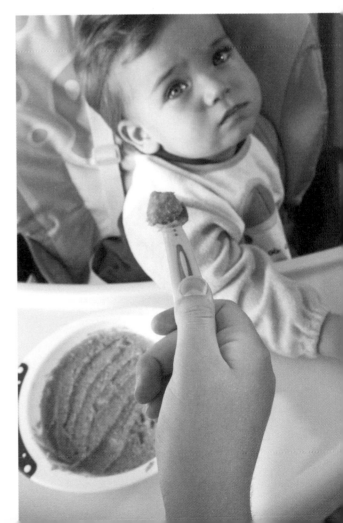

Only a small percentage of children have serious problems eating and it is nearly always down to behaviour. Others may have been premature babies (with feeding tubes or ventilation) and will react to anything touching their lips. Or they may find it hard to co-ordinate sucking and breathing.

I always do a discreet check about feeding styles. Is there anything unconventional about how you feed him? How about your nutritional beliefs? Could control be an issue – for you or for him?

Home Treatment: Refusing to Eat

Don't force him to eat. He won't starve and tension will only make things worse. Try to be creative instead. His diet can be narrower than you would like – just as long as he is gaining weight and is getting the vitamins and minerals he needs.

- **Draw a circle** around the foods on offer (the healthy range). Then you can be more flexible about what – and even when – he eats.

- **Don't insist on three formal meals.** Your child can reach his daily food target by grazing – as long as the snacks and drinks are healthy (fruit, cheese, milk, sandwiches).

- **Always nudge his limits** with new foods. Start with tiny tastes.

- **Aim for a wide choice of food.** But if he'll only eat pancakes and chicken, that's fine. It is boring but healthy (sneak a little chopped carrot in) and he will eventually try something new.

- **Hide meat** if need be in Bolognese sauce or chop it very small. Most children like pasta, bread and cereals and they'll give his diet a solid base.

- **Watch his milk.** If your child is a toddler or older, watch how much he drinks. Maybe it is too much and is filling him up. He does need calcium, though. Milk is a good source, but so are yoghurts and cheese.

- **Vegetables** can be a battle, but soups can work. Fruit can compensate in the meantime, but simply giving him extra fruit juice is not a good idea.

- **Be a little careful with smoothies**, which are now a hot topic. They are not as good as eating fresh fruit. Juicing removes nutrients and fibre and some smoothies are made from concentrate fruit. But if he eats nothing, by all means use them – they are high in calories – but in moderation.

- **Try food games** from the earliest age. Siblings are named after carrot sticks, then gobbled up in turn. Tiny broccoli florets are a magic forest that slowly disappears. After a few runs at it, he may decide to join the game.

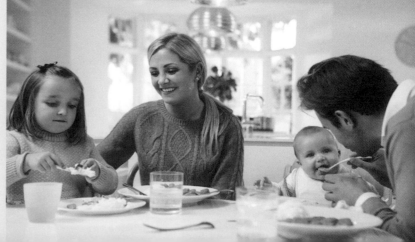

Using food games can encourage children to eat at mealtimes

➕ **If his diet is very narrow**, make sure it includes foods that provide the vitamins and minerals (such as iron) he needs. Fortified cow's milk can be used if he is over one year. But no matter how bad an eater your child is, I would not use vitamin tablets or tonics to compensate – they won't.

You may be less worried if you tot up what he eats and drinks each day – probably more good food than you think. But if your child is not gaining weight, you should talk to your doctor. If eating is a serious problem, a specialist feeding clinic will help. (See also Eating Disorders, page 283).

ANAEMIA is a very real problem. Lack of iron can affect your child's brain development and it may not be reversible. Yet up to 10 per cent of children under two years can have iron-deficient anaemia.

💼 Is he tense, withdrawn and anxious?

💼 Is he a baby and on a diet of cow's milk?

💼 Does he eat no meat, fish or other iron-rich foods?

💼 Is he a toddler or older and drinking too much cow's milk?

Mood in itself is not a symptom of anaemia, but coupled with a poor diet it could be. Your doctor will do a blood test to check his haemoglobin and iron stores (ferritin level). Low-income families are most at risk, but so are children who drink too much cow's milk, because there is less room for other iron-rich foods.

There are two types of iron in foods: haem and non-haem. Haem iron is in flesh foods (e.g. chicken, red meat and fish) and non-haem iron is in plant foods (e.g. cereals, some vegetables and wholegrain bread). The body will absorb haem iron better, but eating a food with vitamin C in the same meal will improve his absorption of non-haem iron.

Home Treatment: Anaemia

You need to work with your doctor if it's anaemia.

- **A three-month trial of iron** should improve his mood and haemoglobin count very quickly.
- **Look at his diet too.** He shouldn't stay on iron treatment indefinitely, so make sure he gets all the iron he needs from food. Haem iron comes from many standard foods, especially meat and fish. He'll get iron from other non-haem foods too, especially vegetables and cereals. But he will need vitamin C to absorb it, so don't forget the fruit.
- **Milk.** Make sure he is not filling up on cow's milk.

MILK ALLERGY OR LACTOSE INTOLERANCE These are not nearly as common as people think – they affect some three per cent of children.

Milk allergy symptoms can include:

- Crying within an hour of feeding.
- Vomiting and diarrhoea.
- Chest problems and runny nose.
- Skin reactions.
- Swelling around the eyes.
- Tiny flecks of blood in his stools.

If the child is allergic to cow's milk protein, the symptoms will disappear **completely** when you remove milk from the diet – and reappear if you use it again.

Lactose intolerance is not permanent; it usually lasts a few weeks. You will notice:

- Watery, loose bowel motions.
- A swollen stomach.
- Poor weight gain.
- A red bottom caused by acid in his stools.

(See also Chapter 10, Food Allergy.)

Home Treatment: Milk Allergy

Your doctor will help you to test him for milk allergy.

With cow's milk allergy, a trial exclusion of cow's milk protein may work and he will switch to hypoallergenic milk formula. Switching to soya or goat's milk will not solve the problem, as both contain proteins quite similar to cow's milk protein. If your child is lactose intolerant, the answer is lactose-free milk for a few weeks – then he can return to his usual formula. Soya-based formula can be used, but not for babies under six months. I do not recommend goat's milk for babies. There is no reason to exclude milk from the diet in the long term.

The Inside Track

Breast milk

Formula milks have come a long way, but really cannot match breast milk. It is the perfect growth potion and gives instant immunity at birth. Breast milk in his first five days of life contains colostrum, which is particularly high in goodies. If you can breastfeed, he will have everything he needs – whey proteins, fat and essential fatty acids, and carbohydrate. This is why exclusive breastfeeding for the first six months is always recommended. Sadly, fewer than 50 per cent of mothers breastfeed and even fewer keep it up for six months. It is a personal choice, but choosing not to breastfeed is very often down to lack of support.

Formula milks

These are made from modified cow's milk and you will find a confusion of them in the shops. Marketing has quite a lot to do with it. In fact, if baby is quite happy with his first milk there is no reason why he should move on to another.

Chopping and changing milks is not a good idea.

* 'First milks' are for babies who are not breastfed. They are high in whey and the milk has been modified to mimic breast milk. The whey to casein ratio is 60:40.

* 'Second milks' are marketed for the hungrier baby. These are higher in casein (the whey to casein ratio is 20:80) and are more like full-cream cow's milk. Casein is harder for a baby to digest so it is not advised for babies less than six weeks old.

* 'Follow-on milk' has extra minerals and vitamins, and is marketed for the older baby, over six months old. It has been created to discourage mothers from giving pure cow's milk to their babies before their first birthday.

* 'Special formulas' are for babies with problems. Pre-term or low-growth babies will be fed high-calorie milks. Thickened feeds are marketed for refluxing babies – the milk looks normal when made up but thickens when it reaches the stomach acid. (Whether it helps greatly is debatable.) There are also formulas that do not contain either cow's milk protein or lactose.

Is He Getting Enough Milk?

Formula feeding is easier to measure, but there are rules of thumb for breastfeeding:

* He returned to his birth weight by two weeks old and then gained 150 to 200 grams a week for three months.

* He has more than five wet nappies a day.

* His bowel motions are normal (often quite runny).

* He attaches to the breast well, with his mouth covering the whole nipple and nearly all of the brown area.

Your breastfed baby will decide how much he needs – and drink accordingly.

It is really important to stay away from formula milk supplements when you are in the early stages of breastfeeding. It can undermine confidence in your own talents.

FORMULA FEEDING (1 FLUID OZ = 30 ML)

Age	Amount of Milk	Number of Feeds a Day
1–2 weeks	60 ml	7–8
2–6 weeks	90–120 ml	6
2 months	120–180 ml	5–6
3 months	180–210 ml	5
6 months	210–240 ml	4

Is He Getting Enough Solids?

He should not need to start solid foods until he is four to six months old. His first solids should be foods containing iron, as his body's stores of iron start to reduce at this stage.

4 TO 6 MONTHS Begin with small spoonfuls of puréed carrot or gluten-free cereals such as baby rice, mixed with his usual breast or formula milk (it will be runny like yoghurt). If this works well, add puréed fruit or vegetables. Then try puréed meat. It is best to introduce one food at a time, with a day or two between. He can start drinking his formula milk from a cup from six months and gradually use the bottle less.

BY 7 OR 8 MONTHS He should have three solid meals a day. He will also be drinking either breast milk or formula milk (ideally from a beaker or cup). He will start eating lumpy – and then chopped or mashed – food.

By his first birthday, he will be eating the same food (a smaller quantity!) as the rest of the family. He should not drink low-fat milk products until he is two years old.

1 TO 2 YEARS He needs more fat and less fibre than older children (in fact, he will get all the fibre he needs from cereals, fruit and vegetables). His three main meals will be small, so he will need a snack in between (fruit, crackers, raisins or yoghurts and milk).

2 TO 5 YEARS The diet will be changing to a lower-fat, higher-fibre one. If he is eating properly he will have:

- Bread, rice, pasta, cereals or potatoes at every meal.
- Fruit or vegetables at every meal.
- Milk, cheese or yoghurt three times a day.
- Meat, fish, eggs or nuts at least twice a day.
- Six to eight glasses of fluid every day.

RECOMMENDED DAILY PORTIONS OF EACH FOOD GROUP

	1–3 years	3–5 years
Starch	**4 portions**	**4–6+ portions**
Bread	½–1 slice	1 small slice
Cereal	1–2 tablespoons	2–3 tablespoons
Weetabix	½–1 biscuit	1½ biscuits
Potatoes, mashed	½–1 scoop	1–1½ scoops
Potatoes, boiled	½–1 potato	1–1½ potatoes
Cooked rice or pasta	1–2 tablespoons	2–3 tablespoons
Fruit and vegetables	**2–4 portions**	**4+ portions**
Apple/pear/banana	½ fruit	1 small fruit
Plum/kiwi/mandarin	½–1 fruit	1 fruit
Grapes	6–8	12
Strawberries	4	6
Tinned fruit	1 tablespoon	2 tablespoons
Carrots	½ carrot (1 tablespoon)	1 small carrot (2 tablespoons)
Other vegetables	1 tablespoon, cooked	1 tablespoon, cooked
Salad vegetables	2 tablespoons	3 tablespoons
Tomato	2 cherry/½ tomato	3 cherry/1 small tomato
Vegetable soup	1 small bowl	1 bowl
Dairy	**3 portions**	**3 portions**
Cheese	30g in cubes or grated (about the size of a matchbox)	
Milk	200ml	200ml
Yoghurt	1 pot (25g)	1 pot (125g)

Protein	2 portions	2 portions
Minced meat	1–1½ tablespoons	2–3 tablespoons
Meat	½–1 slice	1–2 slices
Fish fillet	¼–½ small fillet	½–1 small fillet
Fish fingers/sausages	1–2	2–3
Eggs	½–1	1
Beans/lentils	1–2 tablespoons	2–3 tablespoons
Quorn/TVP	30–60g	60g
Smooth peanut butter	1–2 tablespoons	2 tablespoons
Fatty and sugary foods	Sparingly	Sparingly
Sweets, crisps, fizzy drinks, biscuits, cakes, confectionery, takeaways, fried foods	Occasionally	

Source: Feed Your Child Well, written by dieticians at the Children's University Hospital, Temple Street, Dublin.

Baby Feeding

🐻 Don't feed cow's milk – or goat, soya or rice milk – to a baby under one year. Your child needs iron to help his brain develop and he will get it from either breast or formula milk. And don't put him on a special formula milk without medical advice.

🐻 If he is breastfed, he doesn't need formula feeds to supplement his diet. He is self-regulating and will drink what his body needs.

🐻 Fruit juice should never be a substitute for breast or formula milk. Between milk feeds, the best drink is cooled boiled water.

🐻 I do not advise giving babies tea, mineral water or fizzy drinks.

Red Alert

TALK TO YOUR DOCTOR IF:

➕ His nappies are not very wet, he is lethargic or very fretful or if he doesn't seem to be swallowing when he breastfeeds.

➕ He seems to have lost a lot of weight (over 8 per cent of his birth weight).

➕ You are breastfeeding and have sore nipples or engorged breasts (after the first week).

➕ Your child is pre-teen and you suspect an eating disorder. (See Eating Disorders, page 283.)

GET EMERGENCY HELP IF:

➕ There are signs of severe reflux: he's vomiting full feeds, very irritable and not gaining weight.

➕ His vomit is grass green (his bowel may be blocked).

➕ The vomiting is dramatic and can hit a wall a few feet away (it may be pyloric stenosis).

➕ He is a baby and there are signs of gastroenteritis (vomiting and diarrhoea with a temperature).

Chapter 8
Fever

'At 6 o'clock, she refused her dinner. She seemed tired and wanted to stay on my lap so we brought her up to bed early and took her temperature (which was 38.2°C). We gave her some medicine, which seemed to bring it down, and she fell asleep. At 1 a.m. we checked her and she was much hotter. Her temperature was 39.1°C. We really didn't want to bother a doctor at that time of the night but we were very worried.'

It's a Symptom, Not a Cause

You may know the situation. The thermometer tells you that she is 39°C, too hot, that something is badly wrong, yet she lies on the sofa happily squinting at the television. Meanwhile, you push work deadlines to the back of your mind. Should you call the doctor?

A high temperature can be one of the hardest symptoms to call. How many busy doctors sigh as they see 'yet another' child with a fever? And how many parents hover over the telephone as the thermometer rises? It is a little like an airport security X-ray: the vast majority of suitcases passing through are harmless. Likewise, most children with a temperature have a simple viral infection. But you need to be alert to the exception.

One thing is certain. Your child is absolutely certain to get a fever. After all, the average child will have some six to eight viral infections in her pre-school years.

- In most cases, a temperature is not a cause for alarm.
- It's a very useful symptom that something is wrong.
- It prompts you to watch carefully for other (more specific) signs of illness.
- A fever alone will not kill her.

I tend not to worry about a child with a temperature who is smiling.

BUT

If your child under two months has a temperature, she should see a doctor immediately.

Is It a Fever?

- An arbitrary definition of fever is a temperature of 38°C or over.
- When your toddler goes very quiet and feels hot to touch, you really need to check her temperature.
- The biggest decision is always whether or not to call the doctor. Nothing substitutes for a doctor's expertise, but I'm a great believer in the instincts of a smart parent. When a mother tells me she is very worried about her child, I get worried.

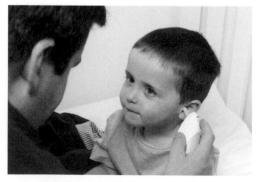

Check your child's temperature if you're concerned about a fever

(See Using Thermometers, page 95.)

The Viral Illness 'Excuse'

You bundle your feverish child into the car only to learn from the doctor that she has a 'viral illness that will pass'. Some parents suspect that this is a medical excuse for 'cause unknown'. In reality, many fevers **are** caused by a viral illness – one of any hundred or so that can rarely be identified outside a laboratory. In most cases, the illness will disappear of its own accord, provided you control the temperature.

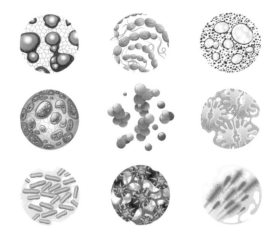

Many viruses can only be identified in a laboratory

Is It a Serious Infection?

There is a measure used in paediatric medicine – the 'traffic-light' system – to decide if a feverish child is at low, medium or high risk of having a serious bacterial illness. (See the Traffic Lights chart on the next page.)

Where is your child on the chart? If her symptoms are amber or red, you need medical help. Go by your instincts if you cannot make up your mind.

A very small number (up to 3 per cent) of children reaching hospital with a temperature will have a serious bacterial illness. Thanks to vaccination, almost no child in our part of the world will die of a serious infection nowadays (meningitis being the rare exception).

Traffic Lights

When she has a fever, how likely is it to be a serious illness?

GREEN – LOW RISK	AMBER – INTERMEDIATE RISK	RED – HIGH RISK
Colour	**Colour**	**Colour**
The skin, lips and tongue are normal colour	She is pale	She is pale or mottled or ashen or blue
Activity	**Activity**	**Activity**
She reacts normally to you She is content, smiles She stays awake or wakes quickly Strong, normal cry or not crying	She is not reacting normally to you She wakes only after a lot of stimulation She is less active No smile	She doesn't react to you You can't rouse her – or if you do she doesn't stay awake She has a weak, high-pitched or continuous cry
Hydration	**Breathing**	**Breathing**
Normal skin and eyes Her lips are moist	The nostrils are flared She's breathing quickly: 🧰 over 50 breaths a minute (age 6–12 months) 🧰 over 40 breaths a minute (age over 12 months)	She's grunting She's breathing fast: over 60 breaths a minute Her chest is pulled in (moderately or severely)
Other	**Hydration**	**Hydration**
She has none of the amber or red symptoms	Her tongue and lips are dry If a baby, she's not feeding well When you squeeze her big toe, it goes white but does not return to its normal colour within three seconds (capillary refill time) She is urinating less	If you pinch her skin, it stays up (like a tent) and doesn't return to normal
	Other	**Other**
	She has had a fever for over five days Limb or joint swelling She cannot stand (or is limping) A new lump has appeared	She has a temperature over 38°C (if age 0–3 months) She has a temperature over 39°C (if age 3–6 months) There is a rash that doesn't disappear when pressed She's a baby and has a bulging fontanelle (forehead) She has a stiff neck She has a fit that lasts more than 20 minutes She has fits on one side of the body There is weakness on one side of the body She has vomit that is bile-stained

Source: Based on the NICE Guidelines 2013.

Is It Meningitis?

This can be a little scary, but remember that meningitis is rare. Fewer than 1 in 1,000 children arriving in hospital with a fever develops meningococcal disease. (Not so many when you consider that most feverish children **don't** end up in hospital.)

The problem for family doctors is that early meningitis can be hard to distinguish from a viral illness – the common cause of fever. They see viral illnesses daily, but may see a case of meningitis, at most, every ten years. Most doctors now keep pre-loaded penicillin for suspected cases.

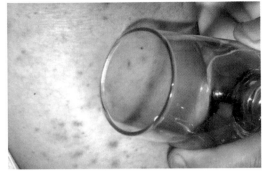

Meningitis rash

When your child has a temperature, always examine her for rashes, as a precaution. As I tell trainee doctors, 'eyeballing' is not enough – examine the whole body. Look in the nappy area and at the feet, as some rashes may show in these areas only. A meningitis rash has flat, 'non-blanching' spots – they **don't fade** when you press the base of a drinking glass against them. It is most unlikely to be meningitis if a rash is confined to the head, neck and upper trunk.

Don't wait for a crisis – practise the glass test now.

A rash is not the only sign of meningitis. In fact, there may be no rash at all at first and (just to make it really difficult) up to 20 per cent of meningococcal cases don't develop one. If your child has **a number of** these symptoms, you should call your doctor or hospital at once:

- Fever.
- A flat, spotty rash that doesn't fade when pressed.
- Unusual drowsiness.
- Unusual crying.
- Vomiting.
- Cold hands and feet, leg pains and skin colour change.
- (In older children) headache: stiff neck; cannot tolerate bright light.

Small Children Do Have Fits

Sometimes, your small child with a high temperature can have a fit – a febrile convulsion. It is a terrifying experience for parents. You see your child turn very blue, shake dramatically and froth at the mouth. Most parents, very naturally, believe that she is going to die.

It is likely to be a fever fit if:

- Your child has a temperature of over 38.5°C.
- She has a cold or viral infection and has been off colour.

Fever fits are more common, and generally less serious, than you think and she will usually outgrow them.

The Inside Track

Medicine now believes that a fever is not such a bad thing. As a mammal, your child develops a fever to make life uncomfortable for the virus or bacteria in her body. The hypothalamus in the brain controls body temperature and normally it can keep it within a reasonably narrow range. It raises the temperature when the immune system signals that something has infected the body – to help her fight back. But the temperature also makes her uncomfortable and getting it down helps to reduce the discomfort and to restore her appetite.

Home Treatment: Fever

If your child is over two months old and only has a temperature, you can normally treat her at home. But if you're worried, or the symptoms seem to be worsening, a call to the doctor is absolutely the right course to take.

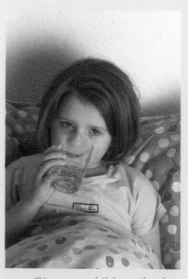

- **Always examine her for a rash**, as a precaution (see photo on the previous page).
- **Lower the temperature with medicine**. Any children's medicine containing paracetamol or ibuprofen should show results within half an hour.
- **Cool her body** by stripping her down to her vest. Try sponging her with a facecloth and lukewarm (not cold!) water.
- **Give her regular, but small, sips of water**. Ice pops can go down easily, too.

Give your child regular, but small, sips of water if she has a temperature

- ➕ **Watch her** for other symptoms and for a temperature rise.
- ➕ **Antibiotics** are not usually needed. A viral illness is most likely and viruses don't respond to them.

Parents are often keen to start their child on a course of antibiotics, just in case it is a bacterial infection. If she has clear symptoms of a bacterial illness (e.g. an ear infection or tonsillitis), I prescribe antibiotics. Giving antibiotics to a child with a fever (but no other symptoms) will not prevent serious illness.

First Aid for Fits

If she has a febrile convulsion, simply:

- ➕ Strip her down to her vest.
- ➕ Lie her on her side in the 'recovery position' (see page 106).
- ➕ Put nothing in the mouth.
- ➕ Sponge her down with lukewarm water.
- ➕ If you have a paracetamol suppository, use it (in the bum only, please).
- ➕ Call the doctor for advice.

The fit is unlikely to last more than five minutes, but if it does you should get emergency help.

Using Thermometers

A rectal temperature is the most accurate of all (closest to body temperature) and is the gold standard in hospitals, but it may not suit every parent. You can, in fact, measure a fever in the mouth, armpit or ear – if you follow the right technique.

However, I advise against using plastic strip or forehead thermometers (liquid crystal), because they are simply not accurate enough. And the glass mercury thermometer is no longer used, because of the risk of mercury exposure.

A temperature of 38°C or more is generally seen as a fever. If you use a digital thermometer, keep spare batteries and remember to turn it on!

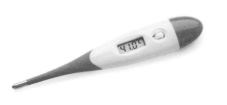

A digital thermometer

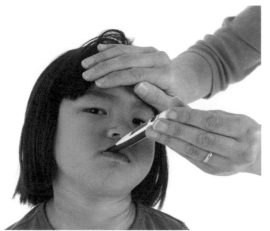

A child having her temperature taken orally

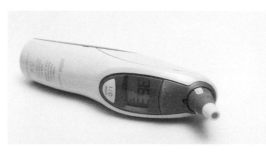

An ear thermometer

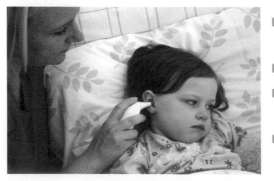

A child having her temperature taken in the ear

ORAL TEMPERATURE This is best confined to children over five years old.

First, clean the thermometer with cool water and soap and rinse it.

- Put the tip under her tongue, near the back. She can hold it between her lips (not her teeth).

- Hold it in her mouth until it bleeps. Most digital thermometers need less than one minute.

- If she has eaten or drunk in the last 30 minutes, it will affect the reading. Use an armpit or ear thermometer instead.

- Don't leave her alone while the thermometer is in her mouth.

ARMPIT TEMPERATURE The reading will be slightly less accurate – around 0.6°C lower than her actual body temperature.

- Put the tip of the thermometer in her armpit (make sure it is dry).

- Hold the thermometer in place for up to 5 minutes – clasp her elbow against her chest.

EAR TEMPERATURE Ear thermometers (tympanic) are easy to operate and are now regularly used in the home. But remember that the reading will be slightly lower than the actual body temperature. You can use it when she is over six months – but under six months it will not be as reliable.

- Pull her outer ear back, then insert the aural thermometer.

- Hold the probe in her ear for about two seconds.

- Disposable tips need to be replaced every time you use it.

- If it is a cold day and she has just come indoors, wait about 15 minutes before you take her temperature.

Q&A

Q **We can only give her the medicine every four hours. What if her temperature doesn't go down in between? Should I give her a cold bath?**

A Every hour of the day, parents phone doctors and hospitals with fears about a feverish child. Many parents resort to panic measures, often causing more harm than good: windows are opened wide and ice-cold cloths are slapped (unnecessarily) against the skin. Others swear by warming the child with extra bedclothes, which simply raises the temperature. Some parents use fans to blow cool air. It's not a good idea, as fans dry the surface water on the skin and so reduce heat convection. Don't panic and certainly don't give her a cold bath. Cool her skin gently by sponging with lukewarm water and stick with the medicine.

Q **Why is 38°C regarded as a normal body temperature?**

A It has been accepted as the average healthy temperature since 1868, when a study of 25,000 patients with temperatures was carried out. There has been some debate since then, especially as the thermometers used were armpit versions and therefore less accurate. It is a useful guide, but I would not take it too rigidly.

Q **Which type of thermometer will give me the most accurate reading?**

A Some people fuss over the merits of different thermometers: rectal versus armpit, ear or forehead. This gives too much importance to the exact temperature level. You can, in fact, use any thermometer; what is important is getting that temperature down. Ear thermometers are quick and accurate these days and are the most practical way of measuring children's temperatures. (See pages 95–96 for information on using thermometers.)

Q **What tests will she have in hospital if they bring her in?**

A Feverish babies are often brought into hospital, to keep a close eye on them and to see how things progress. Tests usually include a blood count, a blood culture and a urine culture. The results will take two days. Some parents are terrified if a lumbar puncture is suggested, but this happens often – especially with small babies – to make sure that meningitis is not a problem. A tiny needle draws a few drops of fluid from her lower back and it is a safe procedure. Within a few hours, you will get an indication that everything is normal, but the culture result will take two days.

Baby Fever

🐻 Be very careful with a baby under two months. They are slow to get a fever, so any rise (or fall) in temperature is very significant. If she has a temperature, phone your doctor **immediately**.

🐻 The chances of serious bacterial infection are very high for babies under two months who have a fever. (It is as high as 25 per cent for babies under two weeks.) A urinary tract infection is the most common. Every house with a small baby should have a home thermometer.

Red Alert

I USUALLY TAKE A CHILD INTO HOSPITAL:

✚ With a fever and a spreading rash.

✚ With a fever and another symptom (such as headache, listlessness, pain, vomiting, poor colour, limping, reaction to bright light, stiff neck).

✚ If the fever has lasted more than four days and is unexplained by any other illness.

✚ If she is under two months old.

✚ I also want to know if she perks up when the temperature comes down. I am concerned if she doesn't.

Chapter 9

Fits & Faints

'She collapsed suddenly during her school prize-giving and it all caused a tremendous fuss. There was no warning; she slumped to the ground and went really pale. I didn't know if it was just a faint – or maybe some kind of fit.'

Most Fits Are Not Serious

It can be as simple as slipping into a short trance. Or, more worryingly, your child's body starts shaking or jerking and she's completely unaware of you and what she's doing. Parents are understandably terrified by a fit or seizure. Is it epilepsy? Will it damage her brain? How can she live a normal life?

Most fits are not serious. They are more common than you think, and are more likely to be caused by a temperature than epilepsy. She may never have another.

- Small children are prone to fits, but most do not have epilepsy.
- Short fits are not as bad as they look. She will not die or be brain damaged.
- Most children outgrow fits — even epilepsy.
- First aid (when a fit starts) is very important.

One in 20 of us will have a fit at some point. It does not mean that we have epilepsy.

BUT

Get help immediately with a first fit or faint, just in case.

Is It Epilepsy?

Epilepsy comes in different forms, but with children it usually shows up as either 'grand mal' or 'petit mal' fits. It is a chronic condition so fits will be repeated — usually without warning and usually for **no** obvious reason.

A GRAND MAL FIT points to tonic–clonic epilepsy:

- Without warning, she lost consciousness.
- First her body went rigid, and then it started to jerk quickly.
- She did not respond to any shouts or sharp taps.
- She may have stopped breathing for a moment and turned blue.
- She may have bitten her tongue and soiled herself.
- The jerking gradually died down and she went completely limp.
- Her eyes were open all the time.
- The fit probably lasted less than five minutes.

Nearly 80 per cent of children with epilepsy have this type and will, with medication, usually outgrow it in time.

A PETIT MAL FIT will mean childhood absence epilepsy:

- The child lost consciousness very briefly (less than 15 seconds) and maybe you thought she was daydreaming.
- It interrupted an activity – talking, playing, eating.
- She stared, her eyelids flickering, and maybe her eyes drifted up.
- It may have started when she hyperventilated and breathed too fast.
- She can have many attacks a day and you may not even notice them! But if she is not diagnosed, her concentration will be affected and she may have problems at school.

Most children who start these fits under the age of ten will, with medication, outgrow them with no lasting effects. It is often a family trait.

Or she may have **PARTIAL EPILEPSY** (often twitching her face and making strange noises while she is asleep) but this can be controlled until she outgrows it. In most cases, the episodes happen only during sleep. They may start with gurgling sounds from her mouth and develop into a full-blown seizure with thrashing limbs. Most do not need treatment and it is important not to deprive your child of sleep.

'FLYING CORNFLAKES SYNDROME' (juvenile myoclonic epilepsy) is rare and typically begins in early adolescence. You will notice early morning jerks of her head and upper body – often quite violent – but she will be quite conscious. She will eventually start getting fits, usually 'grand mal' and sparked by fatigue, stress or alcohol. She will not, unfortunately, grow out of these and will need lifelong treatment.

After an epileptic fit, your child will not remember anything, so you are her most valuable witness. Your doctor will want to know:

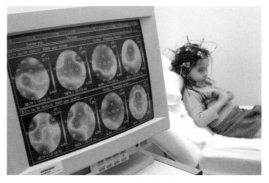

- Where it happened and what she was doing.
- How it began – and ended.
- If she lost consciousness.
- How she moved.
- If she went pale, bit her tongue or soiled herself.
- How long it lasted.

An EEG test can help diagnose epilepsy

It is relatively easy to diagnose. Your doctor will know from the history of the fit itself – epilepsy will have distinctive traits – and from an EEG reading of her brain electricity levels. Your child will not need a brain scan unless something is clearly abnormal or the fits are hard to control – children have to 'earn' scans because of the radiation levels. If a scan is needed, MRI scans are nowadays preferred over CT scans.

The Inside Track

It's not pleasant to watch a seizure. But it is simply a (very brief) brain dysfunction. There has been a sudden surge of electricity in the brain and this has caused temporary chaos – an EEG reading of her brain will show abnormal electrical waves.

Her brain controls her nervous system by sending and receiving electrical signals along the nerves. It is responsible for both voluntary activity (walking, hearing) and involuntary activity (heartbeat). When she has a seizure, an overload of neurons in the cerebral cortex affects voluntary actions. So she seems to be out of control.

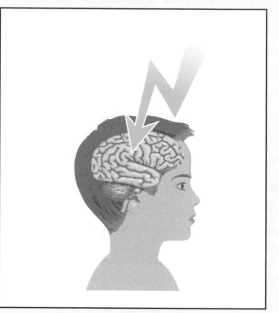

THE BRAIN DURING AN EPILEPTIC FIT

But your child is still the same person she was five minutes before it started – and will be when it all dies down. She is completely unaware of what her body is doing, because she is unconscious.

Anybody can have a fit, if the brain is overcharged (perhaps by a fever or a bang on the head). But it is epilepsy when these seizures recur over a period of time – without any obvious cause. We still do not know why the brain does this, though some forms of epilepsy are linked to genes.

Whatever the cause, an epileptic fit does not strain the heart – no matter how violent it seems. And the brain (though temporarily out of action) does not suffer any lasting effects. There may be exceptions but only if seizures are severe, prolonged and very frequent. That happens very rarely.

One in 200 have epilepsy and up to 80 per cent of children outgrow it.

Home Treatment: Fits and Faints

- **Any first fit or faint** needs an emergency phone call. It is not likely to be serious, but you cannot be sure. But first you have to manage the crisis with a little first aid.

- **Is it a fever fit – or epilepsy?** Try to write down what happened as soon as the fit is over and she is comfortable. It will help to identify it.

- **Any repeat fits** will usually mean a call to your doctor.

When She Has a Fit ...

Phone for help, but also:

- **Lie her in the 'recovery position'** on her side.

- **Put nothing in her mouth**, not even a sip of water.

- **Stretch her neck slightly**, pulling her jaw so that it juts forward (like a goose). This keeps her tongue from falling back.

- **Don't hold her still**. But make sure she is in a safe place.

- **Check her temperature**. If your child is hot, strip her down to her vest and sponge her with warm water. If she has a fever, give her a paracetamol suppository if you have it (no oral medicine).

- **Note the details** What time the fit began and ended, and describe it.

- **Let her sleep** afterwards, as long as she wants to, in any position she likes. Stay with her for 20 minutes after the fit.

- **Reassure any onlookers** It is not serious, she is unconscious and she will be fine when she wakes up.

- **Get emergency help** if it lasts longer than five minutes. Years ago, people held the tongue down during a fit 'in case it was swallowed'. Please do not put anything in her mouth – it may make her vomit and that can be dangerous. Swallowing the tongue is not an issue.

The Recovery Position

Put her on her side as shown below. Her head should be turned to the side. Tilt her head back a little and lift her chin to keep the airways open. Stay with her.

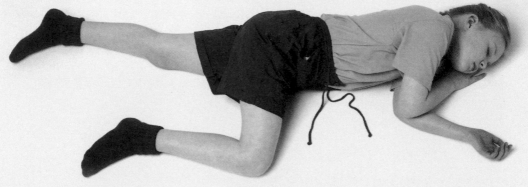

The recovery position

➕ **If it is a first fit**, she will almost certainly be admitted to hospital for observation – and to reassure you. She will have some simple blood tests, an ECG (tracing of the heart) and later, if the hospital staff suspect epilepsy, an EEG brain wave test. Neither a CT brain scan nor an MRI scan is routine, unless it was a complex fit. They will not need to do a lumbar puncture unless there are signs of meningitis.

➕ **If it turns out to be a fever fit**, your child will not need any preventive drugs. If it is epilepsy, she may be prescribed anticonvulsant drugs.

The Recovery Position for Babies Under One Year

Cradle your baby in your arms with her head tilting down. This will stop her breathing in vomit and will keep her airways open.

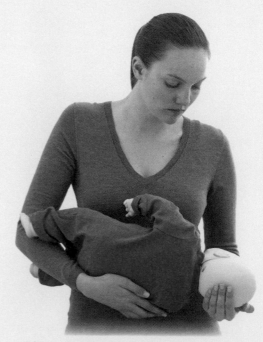

The recovery position for babies under one year

Home Treatment: If Epilepsy is Diagnosed

She should be able to lead a normal life – with medication and a little caution.

- **She will get anticonvulsant drugs** to reduce fits in the future. It is best to take them for at least two years after she is free from fits.

- **Have a home supply** of rectal diazepam or buccal midazolam, to give her when she has a fit. It can help to stop it.

- **There will be some safety rules.** For example, no swimming alone, no locking bathroom doors, no fires without a fireguard, wear a bicycle helmet if cycling and be cautious about busy main roads. It is a good idea for her to wear an epilepsy identity bracelet.

- **But don't overprotect.** Once she is on medication, she can take part in all school and sports activities.

- **She can return to school.** Talk to her school and give them simple, but positive, guidelines on epilepsy. Special schooling may be necessary for a tiny percentage of children (1 per cent).

- **If she is photosensitive**, television or computer games can trigger a fit. If so, she should sit at least three metres away from the screen and the room should be well lit. It is also a good idea to consider special glasses with filtered lenses.

- **Sudden changes of epilepsy drugs** can also be a trigger. If she has to change drugs, wind one drug down and the other up gradually.

- **If she has had night fits** it is best to avoid pillows. Some parents are also reassured by sleep alarms.

- **Surgery for epilepsy** is very rarely advised (only for epilepsy that is difficult to control).

- **A vagal nerve stimulator** (an electrical device that allows a child to 'pulse' herself) is an option if your child is older and fits are hard to control.

- **An epilepsy support group** will be very helpful.

- **Don't stop her medication** until her doctor says she is okay. If you do, the fits could happen again.

- **If the fits are not controlled**, I usually suspect that she's not taking her medication or wonder about the epilepsy diagnosis in the first place. (Complex epilepsy is harder to control completely, but the medication should reduce the fits.)

- **Lifestyle** is unlikely to trigger a fit in a child. But if she is an adolescent, tiredness, alcohol and drugs can trigger one. I would always advise a good sleep routine.

Q&A

Q **What would happen if I don't give her drugs? She's been diagnosed with epilepsy, but I'm not happy about putting a small child on medication that could have side effects. Fits won't harm her and won't she outgrow it all anyway?**

A What is most important here is her safety and the quality of her life. A child with epilepsy takes anticonvulsants because they lower the chances of having fits by changing the electrical activity in her brain. When these drugs were first produced, they brought hope to children whose lives had been severely limited by their condition. Today they allow most epileptics to lead normal lives: around 75 per cent of children treated with the drugs are seizure free.

Your child has probably been prescribed either sodium valproate or carbamazepine, both of which have a long safety record and very few side effects. Sodium valproate has few drawbacks (it sometimes causes drowsiness). Carbamazepine has been used safely for over 30 years and usually has no side effects. A small percentage of children get a rash. Very rarely, it can cause drowsiness, headache and dizziness, but this is less likely if the drug is introduced gradually. If she is a baby and has 'infantile spasms', vigabatrin is usually advised and is very effective. The drawback is the possibility of problems with her peripheral vision. The eyes will need to be monitored while she is on the medication. She will only be given second-line drugs if the standard anticonvulsants do not work well, and these can sometimes cause a rash.

There are far greater problems if your child does **not** take her drugs. She risks having a fit any time without warning. It is very distressing but more importantly she can injure herself. And if her fits are prolonged, they can be potentially dangerous. There is now concern that frequent fits can lead to 'kindling' – that the excessive electrical bursts spark off further fits.

If she takes the medication, she will most likely be completely free from epileptic fits (even if she is unlucky to have complex epilepsy, the drugs will help her quality of life by keeping the level of fits down). She will normally outgrow the epilepsy after about three years and hopefully can wean herself off the drugs.

Q **Her father had epilepsy as a child, so is she likely to get it too? Is there anything I can do to prevent it?**

A This is probably the question I'm most often asked. Is epilepsy hereditary? Yes, it is. Her father will have passed on genes that, if they fall into a certain pattern, will cause her to have epilepsy too. But it is not certain.

If one of you has epilepsy, she is 4 per cent likely to have it; if both of you have it, the chances rise to 10 per cent. What is curious, and unexplained, is the fact that an epileptic mother is more likely to produce an epileptic child. Most of the time, a fit simply happens. There is no warning and – especially with children – no regular 'trigger'. This makes prevention difficult.

Q **My daughter has been diagnosed with epilepsy. How far can she take part in normal sports activities?**

A If her epilepsy is controlled (she does not have seizures), she should be able to take part in sports and other physical activities just like her friends. If she is still having seizures, you may need to take precautions. Do you normally get some warning before a seizure? Reassure yourself that there is somebody present who knows what to do if she has one. I advise a child to participate fully in sports, even if she has epilepsy and seizures, but do assess the risks and decide what is reasonable and safe.

Q **Do computer and television screens spark off epileptic fits?**

A Most children who have epilepsy are not affected by computers or televisions. But with a small percentage (some 5 per cent) a screen can spark off a seizure. It is called photosensitive epilepsy and an EEG will confirm if your child has it. The reaction is to flashing and flickering light at a certain frequency. In fact, she can also react to a strong geometric pattern or to light flickering on water.

If your epileptic child is photosensitive, she can take a number of precautions:

+ Use a liquid crystal display screen (not a plasma screen, and certainly not an old cathode ray tube screen) and reduce the brightness. LCD screens don't flicker and are least likely to cause problems.

+ Avoid widescreen televisions. If the screen is too large, it can cause problems.

+ Covering one eye (with an eye patch) seems to reduce the number of brain cells stimulated by screen flicker.

+ Always watch television in a well-lit room and never sit too close to it. And always use the remote control to turn it on and off.

+ Your photosensitive child may also react to video games, especially if patterns and flickering lights are frequent.

Q Can natural medicine help to control seizures?

A Relaxation therapies can certainly help to reduce stress, which is a potential trigger for adolescents. These would include reflexology, aromatherapy, acupuncture and yoga. But aromatherapy needs a little caution as some oils can actually trigger seizures. There has been renewed interest in the ketogenic diet, a treatment for epilepsy since the 1920s, but only for children who don't respond to epilepsy drugs. It has had some success but the diet is very restrictive and there are concerns about long-term effects, including osteoporosis.

We do not know enough about the effects of complementary medicines on epilepsy. Research is growing but it is still very limited. We do know that some alternative medication can make seizures worse or may affect anticonvulsant drugs that a child is already taking.

I really advise discussing the options with your doctor and making sure that he or she knows if you are mixing medication. It can be confusing for parents and you may find reference websites on natural products and complementary medicine (see page 294) useful.

Most important, remember that if you take your child off anticonvulsant drugs, seizures are likely to start again.

Baby Epilepsy

🐻 Epilepsy is most likely to happen when she is a baby, in the first year. The chances are still high until she is four and then they tail off. If she is prone to fever fits, these will start at around six months old.

🐻 Shuddering spells and jerks (during sleep only) are common in babies and cause no harm. Very rarely, however, a baby between three and six months old can have a cluster of spasms and afterwards is exhausted or distressed. If this happens, try to take a short video on your phone and show your doctor. It will need to be treated promptly.

Red Alert

GET EMERGENCY HELP IF:

➕ Any fit lasts longer than five minutes.

➕ Your baby is under three months old.

➕ It is a first fit.

➕ Otherwise, give first aid help and then call the doctor.

Chapter 10

Food Allergy

'He tried a little scrambled egg, then a rash appeared quite suddenly and now he's covered in red blotches, not just his face. They're obviously itching, because he keeps rubbing his face and it looks a bit of a mess. But he seems perfectly fine otherwise and has no temperature or other symptoms. Except that his eyes seem to be a bit puffy.'

Allergy Epidemic?

Food allergies are having a hard time these days. Ask any doctor and they will tell you that allergy questions from parents are commonplace. Opinion has been very divided. Conventional medicine is full of allergy sceptics – 'We can't really test it,' they complain, 'it's a fad.' Others believe that we are experiencing an allergy epidemic.

I am not a sceptic, far from it: I believe that we have very real problems with food allergy. But many parents blame food for a large number of symptoms when, in fact, the cause often lies elsewhere.

- Many people have minor food intolerances; few have food allergies (some 6 per cent).
- Most children outgrow food allergies by their third birthday.
- There is, as yet, no valid test for food intolerance.

Food allergy is certainly on the rise (in developed and, for the first time, in developing countries). But I'm cautious about overstating the problem. There is an interesting lesson to be learned from the largest study of food allergy to date, the EuroPrevall Study 2015. It found a marked gap between those who think they have a food allergy and those who are clinically diagnosed as allergic. And in 2013 a survey of children's food allergy across 89 countries found a serious lack of quality data. Most of the food allergy statistics were based on self-reporting by parents or children rather than testing. Again, self-reported rates were higher than rates based on actual food testing. Food allergy is certainly a concern, but perhaps the true picture has yet to emerge.

So walk with care when you suspect a food allergy. It may be something else.

Is It a Food Allergy?

Diagnosing is a little like being a detective. Timing is especially interesting. Did the symptoms appear **shortly** after he ate the food? With an allergy, the symptoms will usually show – quite fast – in one of four parts of the body:

SKIN He may have a general blotchy rash, which is itchy. In some cases, there may be swelling or puffiness around the eyes. These signs will appear within minutes or hours of exposure to the food.

GUT His tongue, lips or palate may swell soon after eating the food. He may also vomit, have stomach pain or diarrhoea. The symptoms will, however, be mild.

CHEST If it shows in the chest, it will most likely be a runny (or blocked) nose, sneezing, a cough or a wheeze. Nothing particularly severe. If it is, make sure it is not asthma or allergic rhinitis.

EYE Food intolerance can show up as itchiness around the eyes or as conjunctivitis.

BUT

The symptoms of anaphylaxis are different (see page 121). It needs urgent help.

When making a diagnosis I also need to know:

- 🩹 Which food appears to be responsible?
- 🩹 Was it raw or cooked?
- 🩹 How much was eaten?
- 🩹 What were the symptoms and do they appear each time?
- 🩹 How long since the last allergic reaction?
- 🩹 Is there a family history of food allergy or asthma?
- 🩹 Does skin contact cause a reaction?

If the symptoms are immediate and linked to a certain food, it is usually clear-cut. In some cases, children will come out in a rash if they simply touch the food or rub a small amount on their skin. If it is not clear, I usually advise parents to keep a food diary and to mark when symptoms appear. Your child's medical history is checked; I examine him and do diagnostic tests to make sure there is no other problem. In some cases, I arrange a clinical food challenge. I want to know if it is an allergy or a simply a food intolerance.

Or Something Else?

Food is not always the cause. When his skin reacts, it is more likely to be eczema – especially if there is no early reaction to eating a specific food. The classic signs are a rash that starts on his face and then ends around the elbows, ankles and knees. Sometimes a viral infection causes a rash. But food allergies can make eczema worse and I'll usually test a child under three years old who has severe eczema.

Allergy or Food Intolerance?

You can be pretty sure if your child has a food allergy. Typically, he has his first taste of the food and within minutes his lips and eyes have swollen. The symptoms and timing are usually quite dramatic.

The water gets muddier when (a lesser) food intolerance is suspected. The symptoms may not be so clear, perhaps a stomach that is 'not quite right'. And, unfortunately, no test can confirm intolerance.

This is a problem for medicine, especially when parents expect answers – not a doctor who assumes that they are over-reacting. In fact, we can work together to exclude any serious suspects from a diet.

A food allergy sparks off an abnormal response from the immune system. The body defends itself from what it sees as a harmful substance by producing IgE antibodies (immunoglobin E). But a food intolerance is not an allergy – the immune system is not involved. Your child may simply react to chemicals, either natural chemicals in food (such as strawberries) or chemicals added to food. In most cases, an intolerance is dose-related and he will only react to a large amount of the trigger food. Two strawberries may be fine but a large bowl of them may make him very unhappy.

The Inside Track

Allergy is still not an exact science – this is the problem. But we know that the human immune system has changed. We also know that allergy and affluence are linked, that it is largely a First World problem. Should we be surprised? After all, we are no longer exposed to bacterial illness in the same way as before. Instead, we challenge our bodies with highly processed, chemically treated foods that are still new to the food chain. Our children have bland, simple diets in their first year. Then many are exposed – quite suddenly – to everything a supermarket can throw at them. If we gave them bland diets for longer, would we reduce the level of food allergy? We don't quite know how far these processed foods affect us. We do know that:

* 20 per cent of the population believe they have a food allergy. But only 6 per cent will clinically test as truly allergic.

* Children are more likely to have food allergies (some six in every hundred).

* Most allergies will disappear by the age of three. But if your child has a peanut or gluten allergy, it tends to be a lifelong problem and is potentially very dangerous.

We often do not know why someone reacts to specific foods. But a child who reacts strongly to a food at six months, then avoids it for a year or two will most likely tolerate it in the end. This is because the natural history of any food allergy (except peanuts) is to improve with time. Interestingly enough, he may tolerate the problem food if it's cooked: throwing up a raw egg but happily eating a sponge cake. Cooking reduces the allergic effects of eggs by a startling 70 per cent.

Which Food is the Problem?

Only a few foods account for 90 per cent of food allergies in children: milk, egg, soya, peanuts, tree nuts and seeds, wheat, fish and shellfish. Kiwi allergy is emerging as a new problem (it's an allergy to the protein in kiwi), but it usually affects children who already have allergic tendencies.

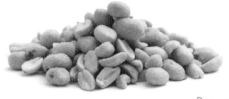

Peanuts

PEANUTS Take peanut allergy very seriously. Peanuts are the most common cause of anaphylaxis leading to death. Unlike other food allergies, this is a often a lifelong problem. (See page 121.)

COW'S MILK The culprit is the protein in milk. The allergy should show up when your child drinks cow's or formula milk for the first time – the protein is in both. He may react in different ways:

- Excessive crying within an hour of feeding.
- Vomiting and diarrhoea.
- Chest problems and runny nose.
- Skin reactions.
- Swelling around the eyes.
- Tiny flecks of blood in the stools.

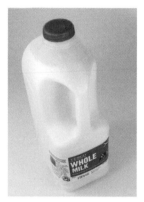

Cow's milk

You know it is an allergy if the symptoms disappear **completely** when you remove cow's milk from the diet – and reappear if you use it again. If he loves yoghurt and cheese made from cow's milk, I usually rule out an allergy.

SOYA MILK People are often surprised to hear of soya milk allergy. If your child is allergic to the protein in cow's milk, he is likely to be allergic to soya milk too – it is a similar protein. The symptoms are very similar to those of cow's milk allergy, as are the tests.

LACTOSE INTOLERANCE Milk itself is not to blame. But your child may lack the enzymes needed to absorb the lactose in milk. You will notice these signs:

- Watery, loose stools.
- A distended stomach.
- Slow weight gain.
- A red bottom caused by acid in his stools.

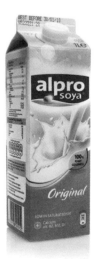

Soya milk

Lactose intolerance rarely shows on its own – it is usually linked to gastroenteritis or another food allergy such as coeliac disease. Your doctor can organise a test of his bowel motion.

EGGS Egg white is the main problem. You will know when he has his first egg, as the symptoms are swift:

- 🩹 A red rash around his mouth within seconds.
- 🩹 Swelling of the mouth shortly afterwards.
- 🩹 A blotchy rash over his face within minutes.
- 🩹 Swelling around the eyes (usually) within minutes.

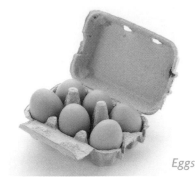
Eggs

The rash may spread to the rest of the body and he may get wheezy and cry. Some children will even react to simple skin contact with an egg.

FISH AND SHELLFISH A reaction to fish will be sudden – you usually know in minutes. He will have:

- 🩹 A rash.
- 🩹 Eyelid swelling.
- 🩹 A wheeze.
- 🩹 Vomiting and diarrhoea.

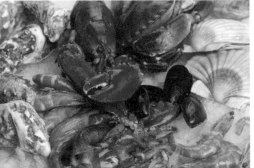
Fish/shellfish

Cod is the biggest offender and shellfish can sometimes cause a very severe reaction. Fish allergy can be lifelong, but anaphylaxis (a severe reaction) is very rare.

WHEAT We are seeing more cases of coeliac disease (about 1 in 300) and I have had three childhood cases in the past five years. It is a very serious allergy, it can be tested (unlike wheat intolerance) and he will always have it. Chronic diarrhoea, not gaining weight and a swollen stomach may point to the possibility.

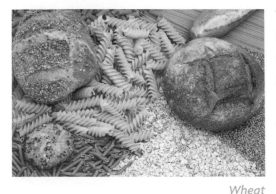
Wheat

This is an allergy to the protein gluten, found in wheat, barley and rye. The allergic reaction is in the small intestine, which becomes smooth so it cannot absorb nutrients. Untreated, the child can resemble a famine victim (pot-bellied and very malnourished). A blood test and intestinal biopsy will confirm the disease and he will be put on a gluten-free diet – for life.

Home Treatment: Food Allergy

Many parents start their children on restrictive diets at a very young age, when it's really not necessary. Worse still, diet limiting has its own risks and can affect their growth. Coconut milk or rice milk, for example, are not nutritionally adequate for a toddler.

- **Don't start any restrictive diet** for your child without some medical advice. Make sure the diagnosis is right before you eliminate foods.

- **Keep a food diary.** If your child is a bit contrary, cries a lot and is wheezy, but has no specific symptoms, it may not be a food problem. Keep a food diary to time the reactions and look for clear symptoms.

- **Then talk to your doctor.** A medical check will rule out anything else.

- **A trial exclusion** will usually put a serious question mark over a specific food. But it must be total exclusion for at least six weeks – make sure the food is not an ingredient in something else he eats (like milk in cheese).

- **Further tests** (such as a clinical food challenge) can be organised by your doctor but often are not necessary. The history of the problem, a good food diary and trial exclusions are usually enough.

- **Milk allergy.** You will need to ban milk and many milk products. Switching your child to soya or goat's milk is not going to solve the problem – the protein in these will affect him too. The only answer is hypoallergenic milk formula (he may not be thrilled by the taste).

- **Soya allergy.** You will need to cut out food that contains soya protein. Not so easy, as many foods now contain soya and it is in most breads.

- **Egg allergy.** Eggs will need to be banned. Be careful, as many manufactured food products (and some fillings in chocolate!) contain egg. The MMR vaccine does not contain eggs (this is a common myth).

- **Wheat gluten allergy (coeliac disease).** He will need to remain on a gluten-free diet for life. Shops and restaurants are now more aware of the problem and can usually offer gluten-free products.

- **Seafood allergy.** Fish and shellfish will be out. But remember that prawns can creep into restaurant (and takeaway) dishes.

- **Probiotics** are often advised to ward off allergies. But the evidence – as recently as 2015 – is not there to support giving them to babies.

- **Immunotherapy** can help pollen allergies but so far has had no effect on food allergy.

- ➕ **Avoid highly processed foods.** Why test your child's ability to tolerate them?
- ➕ If it's food intolerance, **stop the food** and see what happens, but get medical advice. He may grow out of it.
- ➕ **If he has had anaphylaxis**, you cannot take any chances. It means avoiding all foods containing peanuts — which is difficult, as we increasingly find peanuts in manufactured foods such as vegetarian burgers, cake icing, even in skin creams. He will also need to carry a pre-loaded syringe of adrenaline (an Epipen) and everyone must be trained to use it. In fact, very few children will have an Epipen — don't expect one just because he has a food allergy.
- ➕ **Re-test him every 12 months** as many allergies vanish with age.

Q&A

Q Why do so many people seem to have a wheat allergy?

A It's much more likely that they have wheat intolerance, not an allergy — they feel bloated or full. Or the problem may stem from something else. Wheat intolerance is not as common as people think, but it should always be checked out. Some now believe that wheat only seems to cause problems because it's hard to digest in the large amounts we consume today — that it is dose-related. After all, people are now eating twice as much wheat as their parents did. Other studies have suggested that bloating is not, in fact, caused by wheat but by overeating, irregular meals, female hormones or stress-related indigestion. It is still a very unclear area.

Q How good are allergy tests? A skin prick test is appealing, because it's quick and will give me some answers.

A If only there was an easy way to test for food allergy. But if you want any certainty you will need time and a fully controlled test. Your child may be offered a skin prick test or an IgE-specific antibody test, and they can be useful, but both tests have considerable drawbacks — they are not foolproof.

Skin prick tests may tell you if there is an IgE-mediated reaction to a food. A drop of the food as a purified allergen will be injected into his

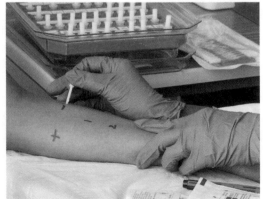

Skinprick testing: a drop of the food is injected into the skin

skin. This creates an antibody, which causes a mark to appear on the skin. The only problem is that false positive and false negative results happen too often. If your child is on steroids or antihistamines when taking the test, it will not be valid at all. Testing is not practical for small infants.

Food-specific IgE tests are blood tests that measure IgE antibodies. They will measure reactions in the blood to a variety of different foods, but the results are also unreliable (for the same reasons). They can help diagnose an allergy, and recovery from an allergy, up to a point. But they cannot be certain.

A food challenge in a hospital or allergy clinic is the ultimate test; the most likely to be fully controlled and accurate.

Q **How about alternative tests?**

A When you start looking beyond hospital allergy tests, the choices multiply. Maybe conventional medicine has shot itself in the foot. When it tests for an allergy it wants to see an immune reaction, the sensitising antibody IgE. This is very specific (and the research is convincing), but it's too narrow for some. So the doors have opened to alternative allergy specialists. Quite a few parents will have tried something from this list:

+ Radionics
+ Pulse testing
+ Enzyme potentiated desensitisation
+ Isolated IgE testing
+ Auricular cardiac reflex testing
+ Applied kinesiology
+ Vega testing
+ Trace metal hair analysis.

Other more adventurous tests include urine therapy, transepidermal desensitisation or rotation diets. And the list — as long as parents go looking for alternatives — is growing.

How will history judge these tests? It is difficult to know, but what would concern me is the fact that many have never been objectively tested. Those that have been tested were found to be of **no value** (except, perhaps, to reassure the parent). More worrying is the fact that some of the more creative tests can be dangerous.

Q   Why do you need a food challenge to confirm a food allergy?

A   The gold standard for testing a food allergy is a food challenge. In a nutshell, it means giving a particular food and seeing if a reaction happens.

Some parents will have tried food challenges at home – taking the food out of their child's diet for a few weeks. Home tests like these can throw a serious question mark over specific foods, but there is always the risk of other medical conditions blurring the situation. A child's diet should only be restricted for very good reasons.

A food challenge is always carried out in a hospital or special clinic with medical supervision, especially where serious allergic reactions are a worry. Your child is tested, fasting, with small amounts of the food that is being tested; or with a placebo – a harmless alternative – to guarantee objective testing. The amount given is doubled every 30 to 60 minutes and he is observed for up to eight hours. The child is monitored very carefully for an anaphylactic reaction to the food, which usually happens within the first two hours.

Q   How do I know if he has outgrown his food allergy?

A   This is not clear-cut. With peanut and gluten allergies, it is an absolute – the allergy is lifelong. But with other foods you will have to re-challenge him at some point and see how he reacts. If he tolerates the food without any problems, let him keep eating it. But if the allergic symptoms return, stop the food for another period. And challenge it again at a later stage.

Baby Allergy

🐻   Some babies just take time adjusting to formula milk. Others will have an allergy to milk. (This means any kind of milk – cow's, goat's or soya bean; fresh and formula.)

🐻   Your baby cannot be allergic to breast milk, but if you are breastfeeding, avoid highly allergenic foods such as peanuts, nuts and seafood yourself. They may affect him.

🐻   Any other food allergies will show up when he starts solids. Don't delay introducing your baby to allergenic foods as it doesn't seem to reduce his chances of allergy. It's now thought that early introduction actually helps tolerance. Start with small tastes and keep an eye out for a reaction. Baking his first eggs or cow's milk may also help.

Red Alert

A DRAMATIC REACTION TO FOOD – ANAPHYLAXIS – IS RARE BUT CAN BE FATAL. LOOK FOR:

- Itching, either in one area or all over his body.
- A strange taste in his mouth.
- Swelling around his mouth and throat and swallowing problems.
- Breathing difficulty and a wheeze.
- A red, blotchy rash like a nettle sting.
- Stomach pain, diarrhoea or vomiting.
- Fainting or a collapse.
- A sense of impending doom ('I feel really strange, scary').

THIS IS URGENT. GET EMERGENCY HELP. STAY WITH YOUR CHILD.

He may not have all of these symptoms, but it's especially worrying if his condition changes dramatically. One mother described it: 'He went deathly white, his eyes puffed up and he had difficulty breathing. We knew that something drastic was happening.' Peanut allergy is the most common cause.

Chapter 11
Gastroenteritis

'Kate woke us all suddenly at 4.30 a.m. by throwing up violently all over her bed. It seemed that every time I changed the sheets, she'd have another bout. Then she started from the other end, to make matters worse. She couldn't keep anything down, not even water.'

Vomiting and Diarrhoea

It starts quite suddenly. Maybe she is a little irritable and off her food, then quite quickly she is firing from both ends. All babies vomit or have diarrhoea, but if she has both together – **and a lot of it** – it is most likely to be acute gastroenteritis.

- It is 80 per cent likely to be a mild virus in the bowel.
- The single biggest risk (and it can be serious) is that she will get dehydrated.
- The best remedy is an oral rehydration solution.
- Starvation is not a good idea.

In most cases, you can handle it at home and it will settle within 48 hours. However, it's important that you talk to your doctor first and keep in touch.

BUT

If your baby is under six months, contact your doctor immediately.

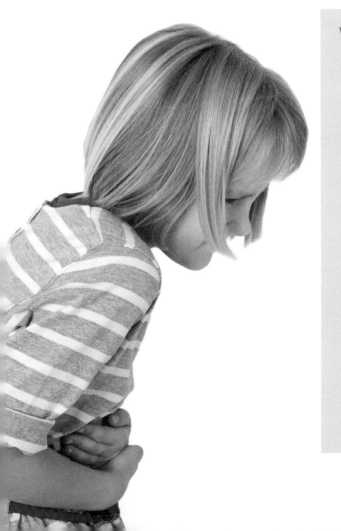

When It's Too Much

How do you judge what is 'normal'? There are generally two scenarios:

Type 1
The child is spewing a little milk (maybe a dessertspoonful) and not only around feeding time. Perhaps her nappies are softer than normal, a curious colour or have bits of undigested food. It's all pretty normal and will generally right itself. Spewing is her way of self-regulating milk intake. Diarrhoea on its own can be sparked by a new food, teething, antibiotics or something that's too sugary or spicy.

Type 2
She is throwing up dramatically more than usual and her nappies are nearly liquid. It's a lot and is almost certainly gastroenteritis.

Is It Gastroenteritis?

It is likely to be gastroenteritis if she **suddenly**:

- Starts vomiting and diarrhoea, with or without nausea.
- Has stomach pains.
- Has a temperature (mild or high).

Or Something Else?

It could be. The problem is that many of the symptoms can be a sign of other serious illnesses.

WHY CHILDREN VOMIT

Main Causes	Other Symptoms
Gastroenteritis (80 per cent)	+ diarrhoea + usually fever
Appendicitis	+ constant stomach pains, which get stronger and last over 4 hours
Blocked intestine	+ vomit is 'grass green' + stomach pains
Pyloric stenosis	+ forceful vomiting in a baby up to three months old (it's dramatic) + vomiting in a young baby that gets steadily worse
Urinary tract infection	+ fever, stomach pains, pain when urinating
Meningitis	+ fever, unusual crying, listless, flat spots which do not fade when pressed

Gastro-oesophageal reflux can cause babies to vomit feeds, because of a weak stomach muscle. Simple reflux is more common than people think and babies do outgrow it. If vomiting is regular and your baby is very cranky and not gaining weight, talk to your doctor.

The Inside Track

Almost every child will have a bout of gastroenteritis before their fifth birthday. It is most likely to be caused by rotavirus, a virus in the bowel. This is an infectious little bug and there is a good chance everyone in the house will get it too (every millilitre of stool contains 1,000 viral particles!). Food poisoning from salmonella bacteria is less likely – if the diarrhoea is bloodstained I would usually test for it. Even rarer in these parts (luckily) is dysentery, a nasty parasite in the gut.

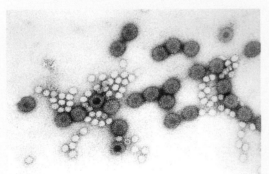

Gastroenteritis is usually caused by rotavirus, a virus in the bowel

Whatever the cause of gastroenteritis, her body will want to eject the alien. So the stomach and bowel empty their contents as quickly as possible through the two exits.

Unfortunately, a lot of the essential body fluids and minerals (sodium, potassium and chloride) get lost along the way. Our bodies are remarkably good at absorbing water – a child will take in more than one litre of fluids a day and yet less than 300 ml will end up down the toilet. But with a gastric bout, a toxin is formed and this floods the bowel with fluid. The resulting diarrhoea can dry her out very quickly.

Every year, millions of small children in developing countries die from gastroenteritis and even in developed countries it can be serious – the problem is always dehydration. In fact, it is the most common reason for admitting children to hospital.

A rotavirus vaccine is now available in most European countries and is reducing winter outbreaks of the bug considerably. In New South Wales the vaccine has halved the number of winter stomach bugs.

The Great Glucose Discovery

It was probably one of the greatest discoveries in children's medicine: glucose can help the body to absorb water and salts quickly. So for millions of children with gastroenteritis, a rehydration drink with glucose could save lives. But – **and this is really important** – a drink with more than 2 per cent glucose has the opposite effect. It floods the bowels with water and actually increases diarrhoea.

The magic glucose dose is now known to be 2 per cent. So do not simply spoon sugar (or salt) into her drink.

The 7Up Myth

If you mention tummy bugs, many parents will think of 7Up. For years, it has been the crude home remedy – a seemingly easy way of giving glucose. It's usually in the house and what child will refuse it?

In fact, you should not give flat 7Up as the glucose concentration is far too high – it's more than three times the safe level if she's sick. Lucozade is even higher, with an 18 per cent glucose concentration. Both may make things worse, by increasing diarrhoea. They also offer the body no salts. Soft drinks, fruit juices and teas are not a good idea for the same reason. As for chicken broth, it is too salty and will also make things worse. The best remedy is an oral rehydration solution.

Rehydration Solutions

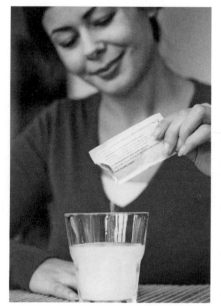

Rehydration solutions are now accepted as the magic remedy for gastroenteritis

Some parents prefer a natural remedy, but this is in fact a powdered mix of natural ingredients. It is simply salt, potassium and small amounts of glucose – with fruit flavourings to make it drinkable. No nasty chemicals and it is drunk diluted with water. The most common rehydration solutions are Dioralyte, Diocalm Junior, Rehidrat, Pedialyte, Infalyte and Electrolade. Oral rehydration was one of the most important medical advances of the 20th century and it has been one of the most frequently tested children's medicines. The modern version has kept millions of children alive and rice-based versions have even been created in some countries.

It is now accepted as the magic remedy for gastroenteritis. It gives the absolute balance of salts and 2 per cent glucose, enough to replace lost fluids but not enough to flood the body. It will work better than any other remedy and speed your child's recovery so that – importantly – she can feed normally within a day. It's not quite as delicious as you would like, but a little patience will get it into her.

The Starvation Myth

The old advice was to 'starve her out of it', but not any more. Without food, diarrhoea tends to last longer and the gut is slower to recover. If you starve your child, she will also lose weight, and that is not good. The same goes for liquid diets over a day or two. Doctors call the nasty results 'starvation stools'.

The sooner she feeds, the better, whether she still has diarrhoea or not. After four hours of the rehydration solution, she can go back to full feeds.

Dehydration

It is very likely that she is dehydrated if she has had liquid nappies more than eight times in a day and has not been treated. Your child could be seriously dehydrated if she is very pale, has sunken eyes, a dry mouth and a fast heartbeat and is very thirsty and listless.

Home Treatment: Gastroenteritis

My advice is to worry less about what is coming out – and more about keeping her drinking. Keep in contact with your doctor and if you're both concerned, she should be seen quickly.

Is it an infection or food poisoning? It is most likely a viral infection, but this home treatment applies to both (you'll know it's a virus if her siblings start vomiting too).

Day One

- **For the first four hours**, give her **nothing** except an oral rehydration solution (and breast milk if you are feeding her yourself). Start her on the solution at once – as soon as the vomiting starts. You can buy it over the counter in a chemist if it is not in your cupboard.

- **Give small spoonfuls every 10 to 15 minutes**. She might not love it, but persevere. A spoon is better than a bottle as you can control what she takes. If she is vomiting it up, start with tiny sips and gradually increase the dose.

- **Make up a covered jug** of the solution and keep it in the fridge (up to 24 hours). Or you can freeze it and give it to her as ice pops. Never add sugar or salt to it.

- **If you can't get the solution**, give her frequent sips of boiled, cooled water. Don't give soft drinks like flat 7Up, fruit juices or herbal teas – they will make things worse. But if she spits everything back at you, resort to using three parts cooled, boiled water to one part lemonade.

- **Some parents try natural remedies**, including ginger and peppermint tea, but an oral hydration solution gives the salt/glucose balance she needs.

- **Keep breastfeeding**, even while she is taking an oral rehydration solution. But stop formula feeds.

- **After four hours** of rehydration solutions, try a little solid food and start her normal formula milk again. Increase her solids if she keeps the food down, but keep it bland (rice, potato, banana, toast, yoghurt, pumpkin, etc.). Raisins are very useful and easy to take, but only for older children. No spicy, oily or sugary foods.

- **If she vomits up the food**, keep her on the solution for up to 24 hours.

- **Keep washing.** Gastroenteritis is infectious, so make sure that everyone's hands are kept washed. Surfaces around her will be dodgy until fully cleaned.

- **Stay with her.** Keep a large bowl beside her and a large towel under her. Or camp in the bathroom until the vomiting eases.

- **It could be a long night**.

Day Two

- **Return to her full diet after 24 hours**, even if she still has diarrhoea. Prolonged starvation isn't a good idea.

- **Diarrhoea may continue for up to two weeks** after the bug (or she may get very constipated) but both are quite normal.

- **Keep her off school** until the vomiting and diarrhoea stop. She is very infectious until then.

Medicines

- **Keep her temperature down** with the normal dose of paracetamol or ibuprofen. If she vomits it up, try sponging her down with lukewarm water, or other fever-reducing methods (see page 94).

- **Don't give medicines that stop diarrhoea** as they are simply not suitable for children.

- **A small number of probiotics** can reduce diarrhoea and may help gastroenteritis (ask your pharmacy which strain), but don't stop using rehydration.

- **She won't need antibiotics** as viruses don't respond to them. They can also make diarrhoea worse.

- **Keep everyone in the house washing their hands**, especially before meals, to reduce chances of spreading the bug. Hand sanitisers can also help.

- **Think ahead.** Stock a rehydration solution in your medicine box.

As for prevention, consider the rotavirus vaccine if it is available and if your child is under two years old (after two it is not effective). It will reduce her chances of getting winter stomach bugs in future. It may already be part of your national vaccination programme.

Q&A

Q A friend suggested that I give her something to stop the diarrhoea. Is it safe?

A No. The current wisdom is that none of the drugs that stop vomiting or diarrhoea should be given to a child with gastroenteritis. They can cause serious side effects. Stick to one medication which is completely safe and will do the trick – an oral rehydration solution.

Q She's thrown up so much that she must be dehydrated. I'd feel more reassured if they put her on a drip at this stage.

A If she has been drinking an oral rehydration solution, it should be enough. Some parents only feel reassured when their child is hanging on a drip, but it's stressful and is usually not necessary. Oral rehydration solutions were developed as a safer and easier alternative to drips and so long as your child is taking it, it should do the trick. It is now the preferred treatment and, in fact, some hospital drips will simply feed the same rehydration solution. Unless the hospital advises a drip, she does not need it.

Q It's over a week since the tummy bug finished and she still has diarrhoea. Could she have lactose intolerance? I hear that some children can develop it after gastroenteritis.

A A stomach bug can really stir up the insides and many children will have diarrhoea even up to two weeks after gastroenteritis. This should not worry you. The chances of her having developed lactose intolerance are very low as it really is quite rare. But if the diarrhoea continues, or if you are still worried, your doctor can arrange a stool test for lactose intolerance. I would not recommend changing her to lactose-free formula milk (or diluted milk) unless she has tested positive.

Q I know there's a tummy bug going round this area. Is there nothing I can do to prevent our whole family from getting it?

A The rotavirus that is likely causing it is very infectious, but you can certainly reduce the risks. It spreads easily by hand, so keep hands well washed – especially after using the toilet, before preparing food or bottles and after changing baby nappies. If you have a baby, sterilising bottles and teats will help to keep germs at bay.

Baby Gastroenteritis

🐻 My biggest concern is always a small child with gastroenteritis. Older children can handle it better. If your baby is under six months and is vomiting with diarrhoea, she **must** see a doctor quickly as there is a higher risk of dehydration. A hospital will be quick to admit her if there are any concerns. If she is over six months, your doctor can advise you if home treatment is enough.

Red Alert

CALL A DOCTOR AT ONCE IF:

- Her vomit is 'grass green'.
- There's blood in her stools.
- She's vomiting, is listless and has flat spots that don't fade when pressed.
- She has vomited more than four times in the past 24 hours and/or has had more than eight liquid nappies (she could be dehydrated).
- Her stomach pain is constant for more than four hours.
- She is under six months old.
- Always get advice if your child has chronic diarrhoea.

Chapter 12

Growth & Puberty Problems

'He's having a difficult time at school because of his size. There's a lot of serious teasing because he's still very short, even though he's thirteen years old. And he gets annihilated on the football pitch. He keeps asking me why he's not growing.'

Shorter by a Head

When he walks down the school path, he is a head shorter than the rest – and it's not funny. But if you look at the other classes it might reassure you a little. There are always a few who lag behind.

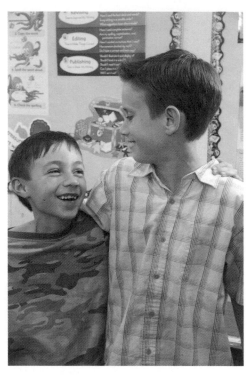

- Most children are short because of a temporary delay in growth. Or because their parents are short (95 per cent).
- Very few (5 per cent) are short because of growth hormone deficiency or other conditions.
- If his **rate of growth** is normal, everything is likely to be normal.
- A **slowing** growth rate is more worrying – I look out for this.

More than likely, he will catch up by puberty unless shortness runs in the family. There is actually little you can do to change his final height – so long as he is feeding and growing at a normal rate.

BUT

Always get a short child checked by the doctor, to make sure that there is no underlying disease.

Is It a Growth or Puberty Problem?

When I see a short child, I am most interested to know:

- Is he growing at a normal rate?
- Does he look normal (his body proportions and physical features)?
- Is he otherwise healthy?

What is important is his growth **rate**. If he is growing at a rate of five centimetres a year, his rate is normal for his age. If he has reached puberty, I would expect it to be nearer to ten centimetres a year for two years. As long as his growth rate is normal, he is very unlikely to have an underlying problem. But if the rate slows down, it is usually significant.

Or Something Else?

It is actually rare (only 5 per cent of short people) to find a medical reason for shortness.

A GENETIC PROBLEM Turner syndrome is rare and affects only girls. Many are just very, very short but look normal. Some have physical differences. They never enter puberty and need specialist help.

A GASTROINTESTINAL CONDITION The classic symptoms of coeliac disease are a starved, bloated abdomen and chronic diarrhoea. With Crohn's disease, there will be diarrhoea and stomach problems. Both affect growth but are quite rare and he'll be obviously unwell.

KIDNEY DISEASE He will usually be sickly and have a history of kidney infections.

HORMONE DEFICIENCY A deficiency (in growth or thyroid hormones) is rare. Delayed growth is the main symptom.

ACHONDROPLASIA is a genetic disorder that's extremely rare. Limbs are usually ultra-short, out of proportion to the rest of the body. Your grandparents may have talked of dwarves.

If his health or diet have been significantly disturbed, it is also very likely to affect his growth.

The Inside Track

Your child grows in small, steady bursts, mostly at night when asleep; maybe a spurt over 24 hours, then a lull for a few weeks. What makes him grow will change over the years:

First year – up to 28 cm

Nearly all his growth depends on food. As long as he's getting enough calories, he will grow normally.

Childhood – average 5 cm a year

Growth now depends on the amount of growth hormones he secretes – it is steadier. Boys and girls grow at the same rate during these years, then sometime between the sixth and eighth birthday you will see a growth spurt.

Puberty – up to 10 cm a year

The sex hormones (oestrogen and testosterone) take over and cause a growth spurt and physical changes. Girls start puberty at around ten or eleven and leave the boys looking very small for a year or two. Their first period is, in fact, the last event of puberty and there is very little growth after that. Boys start puberty late, at twelve or thirteen, but make up for lost time. They often have a short (but bigger) growth spurt and suddenly tower over the girls. All growing stops when the 'epiphyses' fuse; the growth plates in the limbs close and that's it. Girls usually stop growing by sixteen and boys by eighteen at the latest.

Why Growth Seems Slow

NORMAL GROWTH RATE If his rate is normal, growth may simply be delayed – or he comes from a small family.

Short parent: His genes will decide his potential height and your height is a powerful indicator.

Constitutional growth delay: There may be a temporary delay in growth and puberty. Perhaps he is short for his age but medically he checks out well – and is growing at the standard rate (e.g. 5 cm a year). It is really not unusual (they are often called 'late bloomers') and there is no clear reason for it. Around puberty, he will probably have an overnight stretch when the sex hormones start flowing. There is also a chance that he will grow for longer than his friends and catch up. A simple X-ray of his wrist can find his 'bone age': the age at which his growth will stop.

LOW GROWTH RATE If the growth rate has slowed down, there will be a clearer reason for it.

- If he is a baby, it is most likely a nutrition problem.
- If he is older, it may be growth hormone deficiency. But he will be tested for other medical conditions too.
- If puberty is overdue, it is almost always the cause. He's still growing at the childhood rate and needs the pubertal growth spurt.

If there are no previous records of growth, it is important to start tracking it immediately.

Can Growth Hormone Make Him Bigger?

The availability of growth hormone treatment has opened up all kinds of possibilities. Growth hormone instructs muscles and bones to grow and is secreted naturally by the pituitary gland.

This is the master gland that controls the release of most of the body's hormone – those chemical messengers that keep his body functioning normally. They do not come in a steady stream, but in tiny episodic pulses during sleep and exercise.

Since 1985, we have been able to manufacture pure human growth hormones in limitless amounts. It is nearly identical to the natural hormone and up to now it has been given to children with low growth hormone levels (usually by daily injection). It is staggeringly expensive but can bring a child back to his normal growth rate, after a catch-up spurt.

Growth hormone became controversial when the US Food and Drug Administration first approved it for children who **don't** have hormone problems – children who are perfectly healthy, but unusually short (in the 1st centile). It is raising all kinds of ethical issues. Are we moving closer to designing our children? I very much doubt it.

Giving your healthy child growth hormone may cause a growth spurt – but even if he took hormone for 10 years, it might increase his adult height by only 4 cm. As for other effects, manufactured hormone is still young and does not have a long-term safety record.

I would never advise giving growth hormone to a child who is short but normal. It is medically advised in very specific situations:

- ⊞ For a child who has been proved (in hospital tests) to have growth hormone deficiency.
- ⊞ For a girl who has Turner syndrome.
- ⊞ For a child with chronic kidney failure who is not growing well and is waiting to have a kidney transplant.
- ⊞ For a child with the rare Prader-Willi syndrome.

Stages of Puberty

There are wide variations, but girls tend to start puberty around ten or eleven, while boys start later, around twelve or thirteen years old. It is the process of sexual maturing and boys are fertile once they are fully developed while girls are fertile when periods are established. The timing of puberty is influenced by your child's genes, nutrition and ethnic group. The first signs of puberty are developing breasts in girls and growing testicles in boys.

Girls: Breasts develop

Stage 1:   Breasts bud and (with nipples) start to grow.

Stage 2:   Clearer growth of breast and areola (the coloured area around the nipples).

Stage 3:   The nipple and areola now form a second mound above the level of the breast.

Stage 4:   Mature adult breast.

Menstruation starts after a girl's breasts reach stage 3.

Boys: External genitals develop

Stage 1:   Scrotum and testicles get larger. Scrotum reddens and changes texture.

Stage 2:   Penis grows (at first in length). Testicles grow further.

Stage 3:   More penis growth (in breadth too) and glans at tip develops. Testicles and scrotum get larger and skin of scrotum darkens.

Stage 4:   Adult genitals.

Boys and girls: Pubic hair grows

Stage 1:   Sparse growth of straight (or curly) hair in pubic area.

Stage 2:   Pubic hair grows darker, coarser and more curly.

Stage 3:   Adult pubic hair, but still covering a small area.

Stage 4:   Fully adult pubic hair.

Hair also grows in the armpits and on the rest of the body after pubic hair develops.

Other changes in puberty

1.   Boys' voices will deepen and their muscles will develop. Their breasts will normally get larger for a while (even more than a year) and they usually grow facial hair last.

2.   Hormonal changes will affect the skin, especially the face. Inflammation of the sebaceous glands and hair follicles often causes acne in the later stages.

By far the most likely problem is delayed puberty, especially in boys.

Source: Based on the Tanner stages of development of secondary sexual characteristics.

Home Treatment: Growth

- **See your doctor** if he seems to be short for his age. In most cases, there will not be a medical problem but if there is he may be referred to a paediatrician or endocrinologist.

- **Growth hormone** may be prescribed if tests show that his hormone levels are low. It is given as either hormone injections or thyroid hormone tablets. I would strongly advise against giving growth hormone to a short, but otherwise healthy, child.

- **Sex steroids** may be prescribed for a boy if puberty is delayed. He will get a small injection of testosterone to kick-start puberty and give him the growth spurt he needs.

- **Keep your own record** of his height and weight. You can ask your doctor to track his growth accurately over the next 12 months or more using the standard growth charts.

- **Treat him according to his age**, not his size. Tall children are found to mature faster because people give them responsibility. Short children tend to mature more slowly because they're treated as if they were younger.

- **Watch out for bullying** because of his size and talk to his school if necessary.

How to Measure His Growth

The best way to track his rate of growth is using the standard growth chart (see the following pages). You need to measure both height and weight. Mark both with a simple dot, and join the dots to see his growth patterns.

The charts will find his 'centile line' – how he is growing compared to the average boy for his age (the 50 per cent centile line is the average).

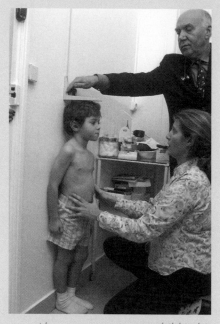

* If he is on the 10th centile, it means that 90 per cent of boys his age are taller and 9 per cent are smaller than him.

* He should be growing at least along the same centile line, or have moved up.

* You can work out how much he has grown in a year to find his growth rate.

* If you have no previous height record, start measuring now. You need to be very accurate and your doctor may be the best person to take the first measurements. Always measure him in his socks.

* Talk to your doctor if growth seems to be out of the normal range or to have slowed.

Always measure your child in his socks to ensure you get an accurate measurement

By the way, tiny or towering does not always mean unhealthy. Some 3 per cent of perfectly healthy children will show below the 3rd centile or above the 97th centile.

The normal range of growth is between the 2nd and 98th percentile, but what is really important is the pattern of growth: he should be moving along the same percentile or close to it.

Track Your Child's Growth

The following charts are based on information published by the Child Growth Foundation.

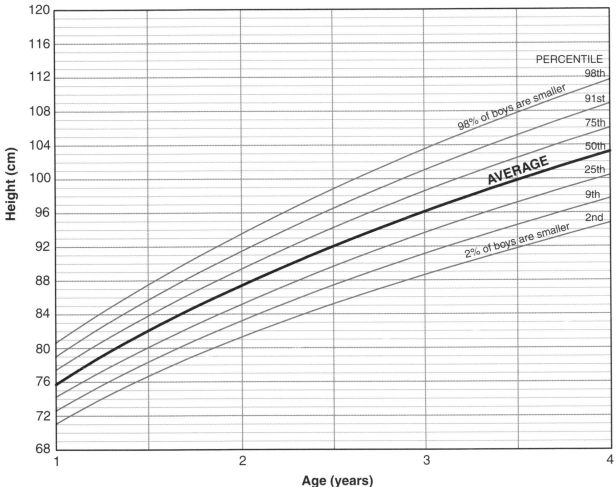

BOYS 1–4 YEARS: HEIGHT

BOYS 1–4 YEARS: WEIGHT

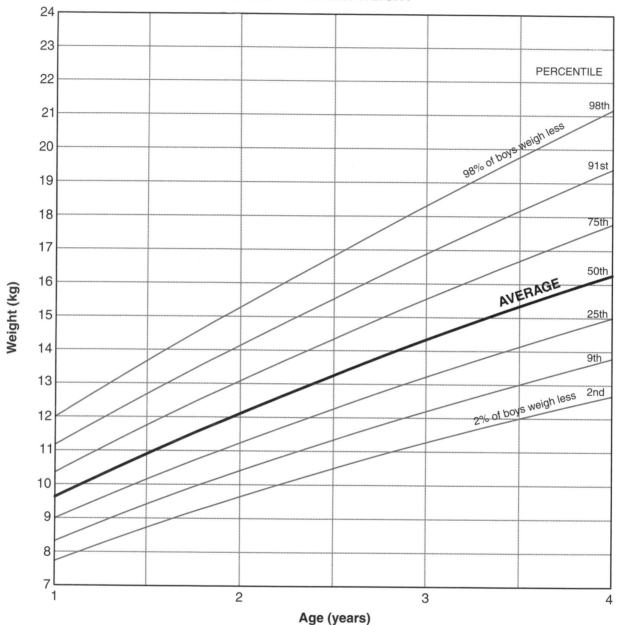

BOYS 4–13 YEARS: HEIGHT AND WEIGHT

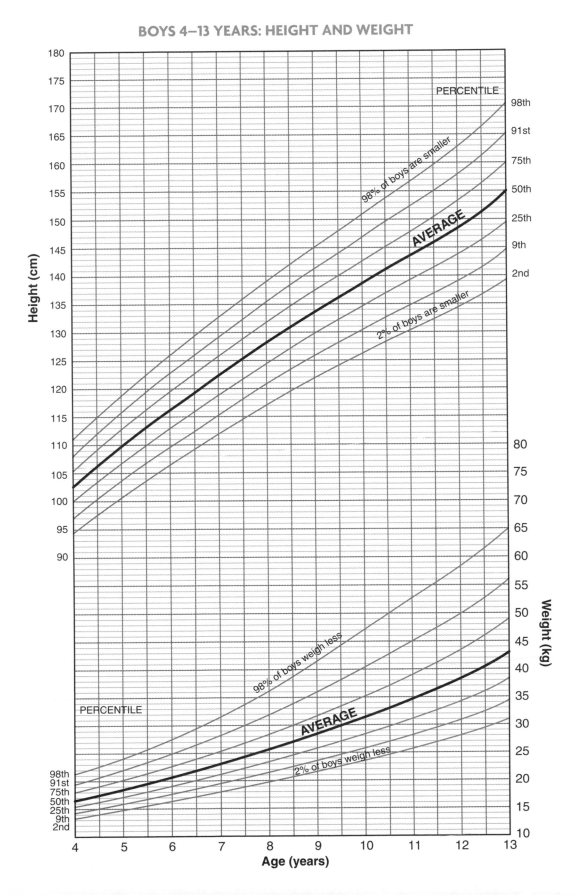

GIRLS 1–4 YEARS: HEIGHT

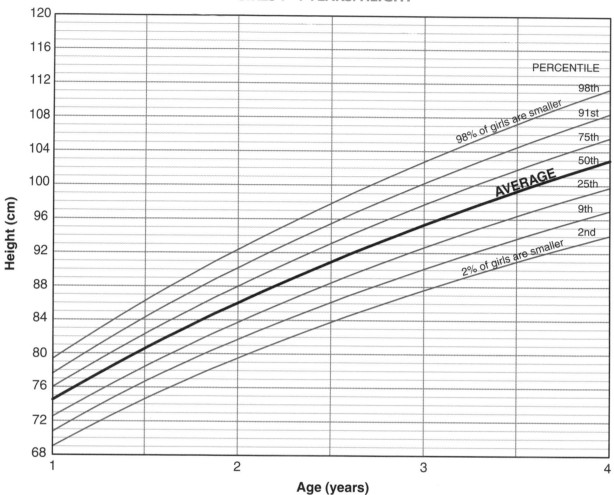

GIRLS 1–4 YEARS: WEIGHT

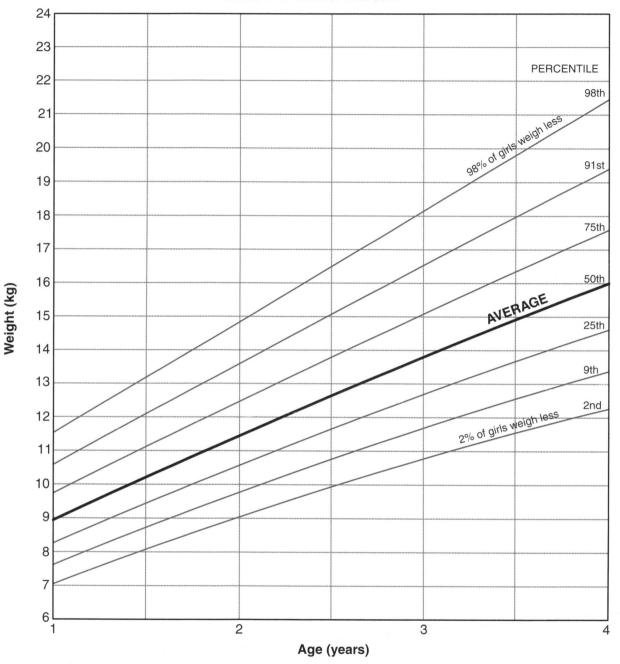

GIRLS 4–13 YEARS: HEIGHT AND WEIGHT

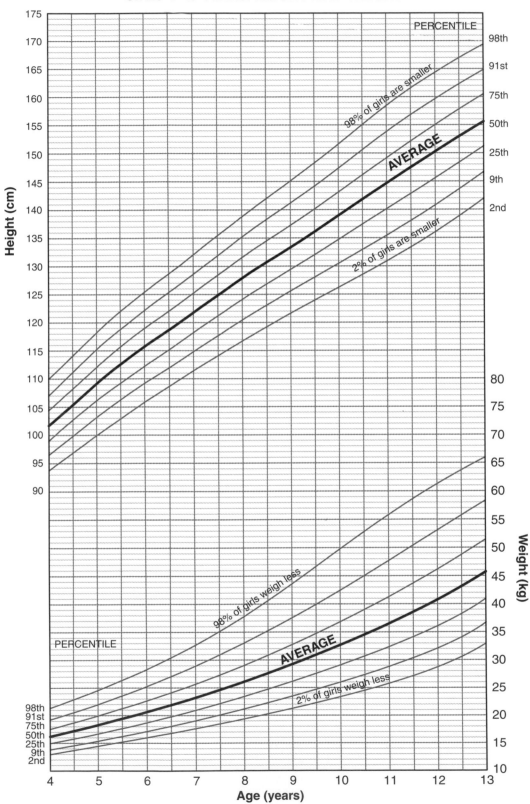

Q&A

Q My nine-year-old daughter may have started her periods. Should I be concerned that it's so early?

A   No. Girls are starting their periods sooner nowadays, usually before they leave primary school. The starting age does vary greatly: anything from eight years up to fourteen years. As her mother, when your own periods started may well be relevant as precocious puberty can run in families. I would only be concerned if she shows signs of puberty (budding breasts or pubic hair) before the age of eight. In that case, a medical problem could be causing her to over-produce hormones. I would also investigate if a boy shows signs of puberty before the age of nine.

Q Why are our children so much taller these days?

A   This is because of improved nutrition in the first two years of their lives – not because of the hamburgers they work through later. Our children have had the benefit of a better diet in infancy and (where breastfed) of their mother's own improved diet. In developed countries, children born now are likely to be three to five centimetres taller as adults than those born 50 years ago.

If you want to make him taller, give him the best possible diet when he is very small. Diet changes when he is older will make less difference to his final adult size.

Q How tall is he likely to grow? Will my own height influence this?

A   Both of your heights as his parents are a very important guide to his eventual height. Small parents tend to have small children and if you are both tall he will be too.

The best predictor is the 'mid-parental height', which is plotted using a formula: If your child is a boy, take father's height in cm + (mother's height in cm + 12.5) divided by two. If a girl, take mother's height in cm + (fathers' height in cm − 12.5) divided by two. But there is also a rough guide. Measure his length at two years of age (at 18 months for a girl) and then double it. It is likely to be his adult size.

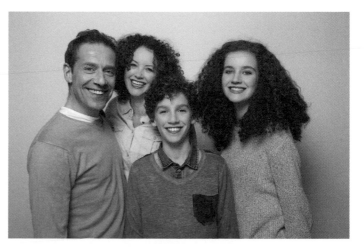

Q **My daughter is now sixteen and, although developed, her periods have not started. Should I be worried?**

A Delayed puberty can also be genetic. But if she is fully grown, she does need to be referred at this age to a doctor or specialist. Stress, thyroid gland problems and a poor appetite with weight loss can all lead to a delay in starting periods. In fact, I normally want to know if a child (boy or girl) is showing no signs of puberty by the time they are fourteen years old.

Q **My teenage son is keen on sports but appears much shorter than his peers. Should I worry?**

A Almost certainly he has constitutional growth delay with delayed puberty. He will lag behind until his hormones kick in and then he should get a growth spurt. When this happens he may grow 10 cm in one year. But do have him checked out by your family doctor and get his height measured accurately. If he is otherwise very healthy, he is likely to catch up once his growth spurt starts – unless, of course, he has small parents.

Baby Growth

 If your child is under one year and growing slowly, poor diet is the most likely reason. You need to look at what he is eating (and you, if you are breastfeeding). But your doctor will always rule out other possibilities.

Chapter 13

Hyperactivity

'He's seven and always in trouble at school for being disruptive and rowdy. He never stops talking in class and can't sit still – his teacher wants to superglue him to his seat. As for school trips, they're a nightmare because he has absolutely no sense of danger. He's likely to run under the bus. It's as bad at home and we're all feeling the strain. Recently he's been wishing he had more friends and was invited to more parties.'

Pushing Your Limit

This can be a very difficult one for families. When your child seems to be out of control and always in trouble, it may test your love to the limits. And he or she will be equally unhappy.

After years of debate, ADHD (attention deficit hyperactivity disorder) is now recognised as a common behavioural disorder and doctors can diagnose it and help him onto a happier path. But remember:

- Not every hyperactive child has ADHD.
- A true diagnosis needs a specialist.
- It is a biological problem, muddied by other factors.
- Medication is **not** the only answer.

We still do not fully understand what causes ADHD but it is certainly not your fault – it is not due to poor parenting. It can store up problems for the future, though, so you need to take all the help you can. Luckily, it can be treated successfully.

Is It ADHD?

Your child's behaviour will make him stand out from the other children; he won't simply be hyperactive or occasionally out of control. If he has ADHD (previously known as ADD), it will be a constant problem that affects his day-to-day life and your whole family.

Everything about his behaviour will be excessive **for his age**:

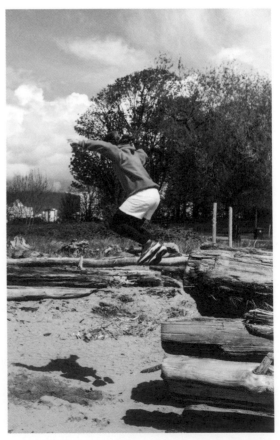

- Inattention (he cannot concentrate).
- Hyperactivity (he is 'turbo-charged' and disorganised).
- Impulsive behaviour.

His schoolwork will be poor, though you know that he is able to do much better. And he may not be popular with his schoolmates or teacher. He will probably be a risk taker and accident-prone (if there is one manhole uncovered in the street, he is sure to find it). If he is in his early teens, he may have become worryingly hostile and even aggressive.

There may have been early signs when he was a toddler (and murmurings from his crèche), but hyperactivity is normal for toddlers and you really cannot diagnose ADHD until a child is over four years old – at least. In fact, I would be wary of a quick diagnosis. A difficult toddler often settles as he matures, especially when he starts the routine life of school.

Or Something Else?

LOOK OUT FOR THE ATTENTION SEEKER He is the child who, for various reasons, mimics some of the behaviours of a child with ADHD. But, unlike the ADHD child, he will usually get on well with his friends and with adults. He is less likely to be isolated. He will probably be as articulate as the rest, while the ADHD child may have learning and speech problems.

COULD HE BE REACTING TO A MAJOR STRESS IN HIS LIFE? It may be within your family or in his social circle at school. If he is a demon at home and a comparative angel at school, it is not ADHD.

THERE COULD BE A PHYSICAL CAUSE An allergic problem like eczema or asthma can make life (and school) very trying. Or maybe he's disrupting the class because he can't hear or see properly? Or because nobody realises that he has dyslexia? Remember that not every child who is impulsive or hyperactive has ADHD.

Diagnosing ADHD

No one has yet proved ADHD in a clinical test. But there is an agreed set of symptoms – the official 2013 ADHD Diagnostic Criteria – which point to it. If he is aged over four and fits these, he can be referred to a paediatrician or child psychologist for further tests.

A. Does he fit either 1 or 2?

1. Inattention

Has he had six or more of these symptoms for at least six months – to an excessive degree for his age?

* Often fails to pay close attention to details and makes careless mistakes.
* Often has difficulty concentrating on tasks or play.
* Often doesn't seem to listen when spoken to directly.
* Often doesn't follow through on instructions and doesn't finish work.
* Often has difficulty organising activities.
* Often avoids anything that involves sustained mental effort.
* Often loses things he needs for tasks or play (pencils or toys).

❂   Often is easily distracted.

❂   Often is forgetful in his daily activities.

2.   **Hyperactivity and Impulsivity**

Has he had six or more of these symptoms for at least six months – to an excessive degree for his age?

Hyperactivity:

❂   Often fidgets and squirms in his seat.

❂   Often leaves his seat when you would expect him to stay seated.

❂   Often runs or climbs in inappropriate situations.

❂   Often has problems quietly playing.

❂   Often is 'on the go' and acts as if he's 'driven by a motor'.

❂   Often talks excessively.

Impulsivity:

❂   Often blurts out answers before the questions are completed.

❂   Often has difficulty waiting in line or waiting his turn.

❂   Often interrupts others (e.g. butts in on conversations or games).

3.   **Or has he symptoms of both?**

B.   **Are the symptoms the same in two or more situations (e.g. at home and at school)?**

C.   **Is it all causing significant problems for him socially and academically?**

D.   **Is there a better explanation – a developmental problem, schizophrenia or other mental issue?**

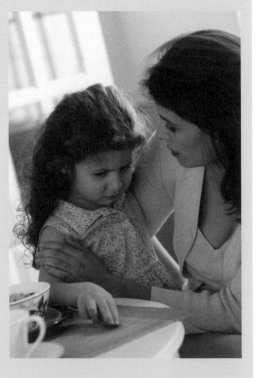

Source: Drawn from the American Psychiatric Association's *Diagnostic and Statistical Manual*, Fifth edition (DSM-5).

If I suspect ADHD, I look at his history and how he is performing in school and — most important — I interview his parents and him. He will be checked against normal child behaviour scales. I also get reports from his school and an educational psychology assessment (and dyslexia test). To rule out other possibilities, he will need a physical examination and both a hearing and a sight test.

The ultimate test is often medication. If he has ADHD, he'll improve miraculously when he takes psychostimulants such as Ritalin. If he doesn't have ADHD, there'll be little change.

The 'Wonder Drugs'

Medication is not assumed and I am concerned that drugs have been thrown excessively at the problem. But they can work wonders for severe cases. It seems to defy logic, giving a hyperactive child the equivalent of 'speed', but psychostimulant drugs do work. They act on the neurotransmitter chemicals that affect the cortex (behaviour control) area of the brain, normalising the chemical balance, so that your child can calm down and focus. Most children will take methylphenidate (e.g. Ritalin) but dexamphetamine is often the fallback. A newer drug, atomoxetine (e.g. Strattera), is now approved in the USA and is having some success. It is not a stimulant and is used in children who don't respond to methylphenidate or who experience side effects from it.

These drugs are not addictive in the doses used. In fact, it has been found that children with ADHD who take these drugs are **less** likely to have drug addiction problems in their teens than those who do not. After 50 years of tests (a good drug trial, by any measure) psychostimulants have a clean safety record. Yes, there are side effects, but by keeping the dose as low as possible they are rare enough. Where they do show, it will most likely be slight insomnia, headache or loss of appetite.

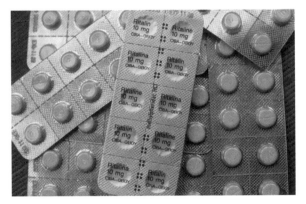

Sometimes the child can lose weight or his growth may slow down, but a change of dose will usually reverse this. A high-calorie breakfast before medication and a later dinner after medication wears off can help. In rare cases, he can get tics and if so, he will be taken off the drugs completely. What happens if he stops taking his medication? The symptoms will return very quickly. Some children can wind the drugs down early, but many need to take them into adulthood.

The Inside Track

When people see ADHD they see a naughty child. A survey in 2007 found that over half of the British public still believed that it was an excuse for bad behaviour and poor parenting. But it's a very real condition. The best parent in the world will struggle if their child has ADHD. That is because he cannot concentrate, or think before he acts, and it is a constant problem. It does not matter how bright he is (his IQ range will be like any other child). If he also has a learning problem – and poor concentration means that up to 40 per cent of children with ADHD do – school can become torture.

Why should one child in a 'normal' family be affected? Surely there are environmental influences? Absent or controlling parents? Food chemicals? These will make his behaviour worse, but they don't appear to cause it. ADHD seems to be part of your child's make-up but despite all the research it's not fully clear why. Or why boys are more likely to have it. We do know that up to 5 per cent of the population can be diagnosed with the condition.

There is now evidence of a biological cause – a slight difference in the workings of the brain. In 2014 the brains of 750 children with and without ADHD were scanned, which revealed a difference in the brain architecture. The cortex area, which controls concentration and inhibition, seems to mature and normalise later in a child with ADHD. It all points to an imbalance of the neurotransmitter chemicals that feed this part of the brain – he will have abnormal levels of dopamine but a deficiency of noradrenaline. But biology is muddied by outside influences: your family situation and your relationship with him, and how his school copes. There are also theories linking pesticides, lead exposure and industrial chemicals, but as yet nothing conclusive.

Can you inherit it? Very much so. I often find that a parent (usually a father) had many of the symptoms as a child. His life – including career – may not have run smoothly and that is an extra complication.

Behaving Very Badly

You need to be especially careful when he reaches his teens. He will be more vulnerable to depression, early school dropout or delinquency problems. If you have other family problems, the risks will be higher.

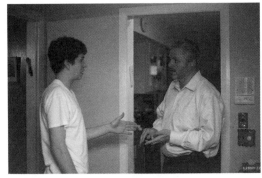

You may find yourself living with a simmering volcano. Unfortunately, up to 50 per cent of teenagers with ADHD will also have 'oppositional defiant disorder' (ODD) or 'conduct disorder' (CD) or both.

With ODD, he will argue all the time and will tend to be very hostile and angry. He will seem to be frustrated by everything and he won't do as well as he should at school. With CD, he will tend to be very aggressive – with people and even animals – and may get a name for himself as a bully. Keeping tabs on him will be hard and he will be the teenager who skips class or stays out at night. It can all go very badly wrong for him. But with help (behaviour therapy works best with ODD and CD) there is a very good chance that he'll settle down by his mid-teens.

Home Treatment: Hyperactivity

Some parents decide to treat the ADHD themselves. But no matter how good a parent you are (or how well informed), some professional help is advised. Remember that he will not simply 'grow out of it'. Behaviour therapy alone might work and all treatments now start with this. If he is over six, he may need a mix of behaviour therapy and medication – with a special programme for his school.

➕ **Get help.** If your child is over four and seems to fit the ADHD diagnostic criteria, see a paediatrician or child psychologist. If his case is complex or hard to diagnose, he may be referred to a child psychiatrist.

1. **Parent training** is your starting point – behavioural parent training with a specialist. You will learn techniques that can help you to handle his behaviour; traditional disciplinary styles simply will not work.

2. **Family therapy** will help to ease any friction at home, especially if his behaviour has got out of hand. You really cannot treat him in isolation from your family.

3. **Cognitive behaviour therapy**, with a specialist, can work if your child is over ten and has serious behaviour problems. It teaches him ways of helping his own self-control.

4. **A school intervention programme** is always important. It will decide how the school approaches his behaviour and also how he learns. It should be individual to him and, ideally, an educational psychologist will be involved. He will probably need remedial teaching too.

5. **Medication is not automatic.** Psychostimulants may be needed, but only if behaviour therapy is not enough. They should only be prescribed if he is formally diagnosed, and he will need behaviour therapy too. I don't advise ADHD medication for a child under six.

6. **Self-esteem.** 'No matter what I do, I'm a loser. And each year the school passes on the news that I'm big trouble.' What can you (and the school) do to help? Is there anything he can succeed at?

7. **Routines.** He will work best when everything is highly organised; where there is minimum noise and distraction; where he is supervised. So he will need routines both at home and in school (and he should sit under his teacher's eye).

8. **Stop seeing him as a 'bold child'.** It is not his fault, or yours.

➕ **One-to-one counselling** by a psychologist is not usually needed. Family therapy has been shown to work better and joining a support group can also help.

➕ **A special diet is not necessary.** It will not transform him (the research just does not back it up). But use your common sense. If the child clearly reacts to certain foods, cut them out. No vitamins or natural products (including omega 3) have been shown to affect ADHD. Herbal teas can, however, help a child to relax.

➕ **Alternative therapies** such as yoga and massage are certainly worth trying, especially if you practise them as a family, though none has yet been shown to control ADHD.

➕ **A good night's sleep** matters, and behavioural sleep intervention has been shown to help. Aerobic exercise before school is also effective.

➕ **'Brain training'** programmes have been tested, to help improve working memory and 'executive functions' (planning and control), but with no great success.

If your child is under four and has ADHD symptoms, a diagnosis is harder. But we would strongly recommend parent training and some form of family therapy to help ease any stress.

ADHD can be treated very successfully. But he will need to stay with the treatment, whatever it is, certainly until his mid-teens. With help, there's a real chance that he will settle down by then.

Q&A

Does he have to take methylphenidate drugs such as Ritalin? It seems to be prescribed automatically these days.

A Can medication help a child with ADHD? Yes, it works extremely well in the short term. Some 85 to 90 per cent of ADHD children who take psychostimulants dramatically improve their behaviour, schoolwork and social life. You'll notice the change almost immediately – within an hour or two. But should every child with ADHD be on medication? Absolutely not. There is a concern that Ritalin is being thrown at too many children with ADHD who do not need it. Or who don't have ADHD. Worryingly, prescriptions of Ritalin have quadrupled over the past ten years as a quick-fix alternative to other therapies. And until recently, most children in the USA aged between four and five who were diagnosed with ADHD were treated only with medication. I'm happier that the first treatment is now behaviour therapy.

Not every child with ADHD needs medication. Parent training and extra help at school can be enough. But if despite these your child is seriously in need of help, medication will work miraculously. A short trial of the drug can often be the best guide. If he improves dramatically, he probably needs it.

Some parents are uncomfortable about using drugs 'to control a child's behaviour'. But doing nothing can be far more damaging, and remember that psychostimulants are not sedatives. They help your child to control his **own** behaviour, because they help him to concentrate and to think before he acts. Simply popping him on drugs is not the answer, though. Medication will only make him less hyperactive and impulsive – dramatically so. You'll have to work as a family to change his behaviour patterns too.

Q **Will he grow out of it?**

A ADHD does tend to continue into adulthood, but with help he may learn to adapt better. Up to 80 per cent will have symptoms as adults – but the symptoms change. There have been studies of children with ADHD in northern Finland as part of a womb-to-adolescence survey of 9,432 children. As they got older, the children became less impulsive and hyperactive. But nearly two-thirds still had serious problems with attention span and were more likely to be underachievers. The risks of substance abuse were higher too. There is good support for children with ADHD these days and you really need to use it.

Q Should I put him on a special diet?

A The diet debate goes on because, in spite of all the studies, it is not clear-cut. Years ago, every child with ADHD seemed to be on a special diet. The idea that food affects behaviour became popular in the early 1970s, when Dr Benjamin Feingold developed a special diet for hyperactive children. Then it was found that it made a difference to only a very small percentage.

A little common sense is useful. All children will react when they overdose on certain foods (the 'hyper' party child). We know that a small percentage of children are extremely sensitive to additives and caffeine – not just children with ADHD. But not all children are. And it has now been shown that (contrary to common belief) sugar does not make children more hyperactive. In fact, researchers now suggest that sugar may even have a slightly calming effect. Energy drinks have been linked to increased hyperactivity in teenagers, but these contain high levels of caffeine. Food does not cause ADHD, but (for a minority) it can make things worse. Changing your child's diet is unlikely to reduce your problems dramatically. I would certainly advise caution with foods containing additives and colourings – they will not do him a lot of good anyway. But don't let diet concerns divert your energies.

Q I've been advised to start him on behaviour therapy. What will it involve?

A Behaviour training is now recognised as an important part of any treatment for ADHD. With some children, it may be enough on its own. With your child, it will try to increase 'wanted' behaviour that is appropriate and to lessen 'unwanted' behaviour. A specialised trainer will help your child to identify his own problem behaviours and to understand both the causes and consequences. Then together they will choose which behaviour he wants to change and will decide on the potential rewards (or penalties). You and his teachers will also be trained to follow the programme that is agreed and to use the same reward system. Most important of all, your child will be taught ways of managing his behaviour. It is time-consuming and needs great consistency from everyone involved with your child – but it can be very effective.

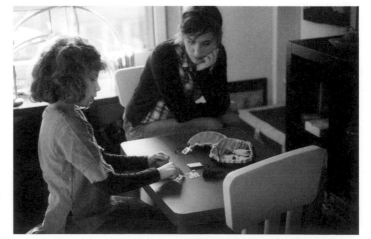

Behaviour therapy is helpful for children with ADHD

Baby Hyperactivity

It is really too early to see any symptoms in a baby.

Survival Tips ...

... for Parents of Children with ADHD

Focus on the positive

* List at least three good things about your child.
* Post them on your refrigerator.
* Celebrate them!

Try to re-direct (not stop) troublesome behaviours

* ADHD children are hyperactive (energetic), impulsive (spontaneous), and have a short attention span (there's so much to do!).

Provide a safe place for free play

Do not expect more than your child can manage

* Avoid too much stimulation.
* Choose childcare that has a low child : adult ratio.
* Avoid formal gatherings, shopping trips or eating out if these are more than he can handle.

Routine, routine, routine

* Meals, toileting, chores and bedtime should be as regular as you can make them.

Catch 'em being good!

* Positive comments should outnumber negative comments by at least 2 : 1 – work towards 4 : 1.
* Tell your child what you like.

Let your child know what you want him to do

* Say 'walk, please' instead of 'don't run'.
* Have a formal programme of positive reinforcement in place at both home and school – use tokens, stickers, even sweets!

Discipline

* Less is more. Make a few clear rules and consistently enforce them.
* Act quickly. Talk (and threaten) less.
* Use non-physical punishment – time-outs (young children) or loss of privileges (older children).

Stretch his attention span

* Reward non-hyperactive behaviour with praise, a thumbs up or a hug.
* Limit play materials available at any one time but change them often.

Communicate daily with your child's teacher

* Work together to make rules and consequences consistent.
* Speak up for your child.
* Teach teachers, family and friends about ADHD.

Refuel – parenting a hyperactive child is hard work

* Arrange some time to be good to yourself.
* Take a break!

Source: Thanks to Sandra Hellerman, CPNP, University of Virginia and Susan Coniglio, MD, Emory University.

Red Alert

TALK TO YOUR DOCTOR IF YOUR CHILD'S BEHAVIOUR REALLY WORRIES YOU. IF HE:

+ Becomes very aggressive or very depressed.
+ Shows symptoms of psychiatric problems or marked anxiety.

Chapter 14

Infectious Diseases

'She was out of sorts yesterday with a temperature and we thought it was simply a cold starting. Now spots have started to appear on her face and stomach so she must have caught something. I don't know if she has chickenpox or if an allergy is causing it. Of course, my real worry is meningitis.'

They Are Inevitable

Brace yourself. Your child is absolutely certain to catch more than one infectious disease before her teens. Most she can live with – generally the list in this chapter.

- If she's healthy, they will usually make her mildly ill at most.
- Some will self-heal and all are easily treated.
- Chickenpox comes with a small health warning.
- Some she will be vaccinated against, because of the dangers (see page 305).

Should you see the doctor? Yes, especially if she has a rash. But if she's infectious it's better to avoid a surgery full of sick and vulnerable people. My advice is always:

- First – phone your doctor.
- Second – see if you can organise a home visit.
- Third – if you can't, see if you can you bring her in at the end of the surgery list.

Remember that the most common reason for a skin rash in a small child is a simple viral infection.

Is It Meningitis?

See page 93.

Is It Roseola?

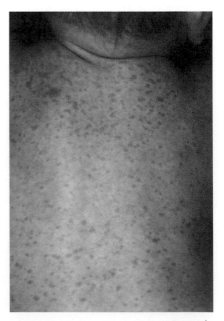

- She will be flaked out and her temperature may put you in a panic, but she will bounce back quickly. It's a viral infection (human herpes virus 6) that is often confused with measles or rubella.
- It is most likely if she is under two years old.
- It starts with a dramatically high temperature (over 39.5°C) for three or four days. It can even last a week.
- She will be very off colour.
- Then the rash appears – usually the day her temperature drops. You will see small (bigger than pinprick) spots that are red or pink and flat.
- Unlike measles and rubella spots, they are quite distinct and do not blend together.
- Unlike meningitis spots, they fade if pressed.

Roseola

- The rash will be mainly on her trunk and neck. It can last for hours – or days!

- She will spread it when she coughs, sneezes or sniffles. It can incubate for up to ten days.

- She may have a fever fit because of the high temperature.

Home Treatment: Roseola

- **Call your doctor** if you suspect roseola.

- **Control her temperature** with paracetamol or ibuprofen. Look out for fever fits.

- **Cool her body** by stripping her down to her vest. Try sponging her with a facecloth and lukewarm water.

- **No antibiotics** are needed.

- **Light food and lots of drinks** are a good idea until the temperature drops.

- **Keep her in bed** until the fever has gone.

- **Wash your hands frequently**, especially after touching her or surfaces near her.

- **If she's a baby** and the soft spot at the front of her head (fontanelle) is bulging or raised, tell the doctor. Her brain may be under pressure.

- **If she has a fever fit** (febrile convulsion), don't panic:

  - Strip her down to her vest.

  - Lie her on her side in the 'recovery position' (see page 106).

  - Put **nothing** in her mouth.

  - Sponge her down with warm water.

  - If you have a paracetamol suppository, use it (in the bum only please).

  - Call the doctor.

  - A fit is unlikely to last more than five minutes, but if it does you should get emergency help.

Is It Chickenpox?

Also known as varicella, chickenpox is caused by a herpes virus and is rarely serious. She is 90 per cent likely to get it before her teens (unless vaccinated) and hopefully she will just feel off colour for a few days. Once the child gets chickenpox, she should be immune for life (there is a 1 in 500 chance of her getting a second bout). The virus will stay in her body and if she is very unlucky it may spark shingles (a nastier, but treatable condition) in later life. The varicella vaccine is now routine in some, but not all, countries.

If it is chickenpox:

- It may have started with a seeming 'cold': a slight temperature, cough and a runny nose.

- Then a rash of spots appears. First you see small, pink spots.

- Unlike meningitis spots, they fade if pressed.

- Some 12 hours later, they become tiny blisters of clear fluid – each like a 'dewdrop on a pink rose petal'. Then they scab over.

- New crops of spots appear over a few days – so she has a mix of red bumps, blisters and scabs at the same time.

- The spots are mainly on her trunk and face but you may find them in her mouth, ears, scalp and eyes. After a few days they spread to her arms and legs.

- Once the blisters appear, it all gets very itchy – especially if she scratches too much.

- She should not feel very ill. Some children get it so mildly that nobody even notices.

- She will spread it through mucus from her eyes, nose or mouth, or a burst scab.

- She is most infectious from two days **before** the rash appears to seven days **after** it appears (or until the last blister has scabbed over).

- In almost all cases, spots appear 11 to 21 days following exposure to chickenpox.

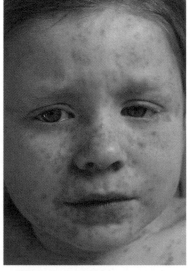

In the early stages of chickenpox, a rash of small, pink spots appears

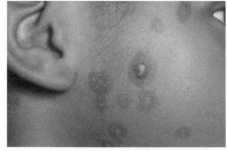

After 12 hours, the chickenpox rash develops into tiny blisters of clear fluid

So by the time you realise it is chickenpox, she may have infected all the family (who are likely to be much spottier than her). The most common complication is bacterial infection of the spots. It can be serious if her immune system is weakened or if it causes septicaemia or pneumonia – but luckily this is rare.

Home Treatment: Chickenpox

Chickenpox is self-healing and your job is simply to make her comfortable. And keep the sores clean.

- **Call your doctor.**
- **Lower any temperature** with paracetamol or ibuprofen (not aspirin).
- **When it itches**, use calamine-impregnated gauze and warm baths. Failing these, try an oral antihistamine.
- **Stop her scratching** the spots as she may infect the skin. Cut her nails to the skin and bath her daily, using separate towels.
- **If there are spots in her mouth** it will hurt. Use paracetamol. If she stops drinking because of the pain, call your doctor.
- **An anti-infection cream** will be prescribed if any spots get infected.
- **Oral acyclovir** should not be given to a healthy child with routine chickenpox. It is for children at risk. (It will not make a huge difference if she is healthy, and it is expensive.)
- **Antibiotics** should not be given, unless the spots get infected.
- **Light food and drinks** are a good idea in the first days, especially if she has a temperature. She does not need to stay in bed.
- **If she wears nappies** and has a lot of blisters on her rear, try leaving nappies off where you can. It will help healing and be less irritating.
- **Wash your hands frequently**, especially after touching blisters.
- **Tell the school** as soon as possible.
- **Keep her off school** until seven days after the rash appeared – or until all the blisters have scabbed over. The scabs are not infectious, so don't worry if she still has a few scabby spots.
- **Do you quarantine her**? She has probably infected most of her friends already. But tell their parents and let them decide.

Is It Impetigo?

This is a common skin infection, caused by bacteria (mainly *Staphylococcus aureus* and group A *Streptococcus*). You see:

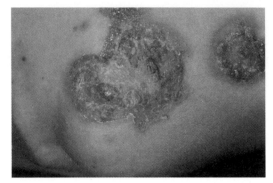

Impetigo

- Small, red pimples that become blisters full of fluid. The skin will be raw-looking and moist until crusty yellow scabs form.

- It looks nastier than it is – there is no pain, it may only itch a little and she should feel perfectly well.

- The rash is mostly on her face (but can be anywhere else). The skin won't scar permanently.

- It's not a 'dirty' problem – it spreads mainly by touching infected children (many of us unknowingly carry it in our skin).

- She will be very infectious until treated with antibiotics for at least 24 hours – or until the scabs are gone.

It can be confused with cold sores – but with cold sores you see clusters of blisters. Impetigo blisters tend to be larger and single.

Home Treatment: Impetigo

- **Call your doctor** if you suspect impetigo.
- **An oral antibiotic** may be needed, if it has taken hold.
- **An antibiotic ointment** may be enough if it has only started. It will also help to stop her infecting everyone. Wipe away any scabs with warm water and pat her skin dry before using it.
- **Clean any infected areas** with soap and water and cover them with an ordinary plaster. This will keep poking fingers away.
- **Wash your hands frequently**, especially after touching her or surfaces near her.
- **Use separate towels** until the blisters heal.
- **Keep her off school** until 24 hours after she has started an oral antibiotic (or until the blisters have healed).

Is It Slapped Cheek Syndrome (Fifth Disease)?

This is a viral infection (parvovirus B19) and most outbreaks are in late winter and early spring. She may feel off colour, but go about her business.

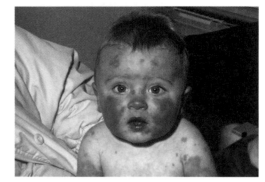

Slapped Cheek Syndrome

➕ She will usually start with a slight temperature, be a bit cranky and her body may ache.

➕ Then the rash appears a few days later. Her cheeks will look as if somebody slapped them – the rash is bright red. If you look very closely, it makes a pattern a bit like lace. There is a pale rim around her mouth.

➕ The rash will often spread to the trunk and limbs and can be uncomfortable.

➕ Some children may be infected but have no symptoms at all, not even the red cheeks.

➕ For a week or two after the infection has gone, the rash can appear again when she is very hot.

➕ She will spread it through mucus – by touch or when she coughs or sneezes.

➕ She is infectious until the rash appears.

➕ If you are pregnant and catch it, it may affect your unborn baby.

Home Treatment: Slapped Cheek Syndrome

➕ **Call your doctor** if you suspect slapped cheek syndrome.

➕ **Control any temperature** with paracetamol or ibuprofen.

➕ **No antibiotics** are needed.

➕ **Staying in bed** is not necessary.

➕ **Keep her off school** until her temperature is down. When the rash appears, the child stops being infectious so she does not need quarantine.

➕ **If you are pregnant**, it is important to tell your doctor.

Is It Scarlet Fever?

This will make her feel much worse, but it's easily treated (gone are the days of fever hospitals, thanks to antibiotics). It is a bacterial infection caused by *Streptococcus*.

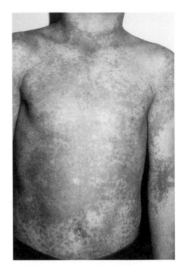

Scarlet fever

- ✚ It often starts suddenly with a sore throat, headache and temperature over 39°C.

- ✚ Then the rash appears about a day later. The spots are red, distinct and very tiny on a generally reddened skin. Her skin will feel like fine sandpaper.

- ✚ The rash will spread everywhere, but it will be most obvious in her groin and under the arms.

- ✚ She will seem to have a white rim around her mouth and nose (a rash-free area) – so clear that you'll see it when you walk through the door.

- ✚ Her tongue will have red spots, first on a white furry base, then on a bright red base (the classic 'strawberry tongue').

- ✚ She will spread it mainly by mucus from her nose or by coughing.

- ✚ She will be infectious for up to five days. If you get her on to penicillin quickly, the risk of infecting everyone reduces.

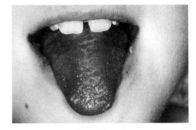

Symptoms of scarlet fever include a pale, white rim around the mouth and red spots on the tongue, known as 'strawberry tongue'

Home Treatment: Scarlet Fever

- ➕ **Call your doctor** if you suspect scarlet fever. Your child needs a prescription for penicillin.
- ➕ **Start the penicillin** as quickly as you can. Nobody else in the family needs to be treated.
- ➕ **Control her temperature** and ease her sore throat with paracetamol.
- ➕ **Cool her body** by stripping her down to her vest. Try sponging her with a facecloth and lukewarm water.
- ➕ **Light food and lots of drinks** are a good idea until the temperature drops.
- ➕ **Keep her in bed** until the fever has gone.
- ➕ **Wash your hands frequently**, especially after touching her or surfaces near her.
- ➕ **Keep her off school** for at least 24 hours after she starts the penicillin.

Is It Herpes (or a Cold Sore)?

Herpes stomatitis is caused by a virus (herpes simplex). It is harmless, but infectious and slow to heal.

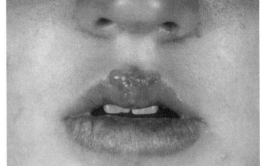

Herpes

- She will have clusters of tiny blisters filled with fluid. Then they open and weep, before crusting over.

- She may have a temperature and be grumpy.

- Herpes usually starts **inside** the mouth or on the tongue. And it hurts like hell.

- The virus then lies dormant in the nerves and can return in some people as cold sores. You will see these **outside** her mouth – around the lips and on any fingers she sucks. Tingling skin is often a warning before the sores appear.

- She will spread the virus by direct skin contact.

- She will be infectious for at least a week after the first sores appear (they can take anything from two days to two weeks to first appear).

Once she gets her first cold sores, they will tend to crop up again, especially when she is rundown or in hot sun.

Home Treatment: Herpes

Herpes sores will die down by themselves. Once they have appeared there is little you can do, except ease the pain. But sometimes you can nip them in the bud.

- **Get in early with 'cold sores'.** As soon as she feels her skin tingle, put acyclovir cream on the affected area.

- **Oral acyclovir** is expensive and only shortens the infection by a day or two, so I do not advise it.

- **Ease the pain.** With cold sores, aloe vera gel or a lump of ice can help. If there are herpes sores inside her mouth, she will be miserable and may refuse to drink. You have to keep her drinking, so give her regular pain relief.

- **No antibiotics** are needed as they will **not** work.

- **Don't kiss or touch her sores** or let anyone else (no goodnight pecks on the cheek while she has them).

- ➕ **Keep toys separate for a few days.** Children (who suck everything) can get herpes from saliva on toys.
- ➕ **Use separate towels** while the sores last.
- ➕ **Wash your hands frequently** when you are around her.
- ➕ **Put sunscreen on her lips** if sun activates sores.
- ➕ **Keep her off school** until the sores or blisters have disappeared. An older child can go back if beyond the nuzzle and toy-sucking age.
- ➕ **Call the doctor** if there are sores near her eye or if it seems infected.

Is It Hand, Foot and Mouth Disease?

This is not as worrying as it sounds and has nothing to do with cows. It is a mild viral infection and she will bounce back quickly:

- ➕ She may be a little off colour at first.
- ➕ Then a rash of single, tiny blisters will appear (they can last for up to a week).
- ➕ They will be small and greyish with a red halo.
- ➕ You will see them in her mouth, on her fingers, the palms of her hands and the soles of her feet.
- ➕ They will hurt in her mouth, especially when she eats or drinks.

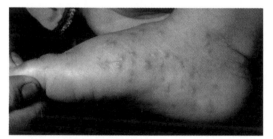

Hand, foot and mouth disease

She will be infectious for a few weeks after the blisters start. They can take up to six days to appear.

Home Treatment: Hand, Foot & Mouth Disease

Hand, foot and mouth disease will self-heal after a week or so.

- ➕ **Avoid spreading it** by making sure that everyone keeps their hands clean – especially after touching her face and hands.
- ➕ **No antibiotics** are needed.
- ➕ **Use separate towels** until the blisters are gone.
- ➕ **Give liquids only or non-spicy foods** while her mouth is sore. Not fruit juice, which is acidic.
- ➕ **She can go to school.**

Is It Molluscum Contagiosum?

This is a harmless skin infection, caused by the pox virus. But it is unsightly and causes a lot of grief. About one-sixth of children get it and it is very slow to disappear. There may be a link with eczema and children with sensitive skin are more likely to have it.

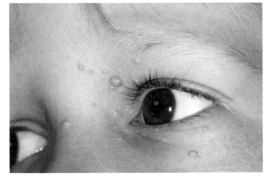

- Your child will have small, dome-shaped bumps on the skin. They are pearl-white and can be as small as a pinhead or several millimetres wide.

- There is often a tiny, hard centre that is indented.

- They appear mainly on her trunk, face and neck.

- The bumps tend not to be sore or itchy. They will not blister or burst.

- She may spread it by direct contact or through towels. But it is not very contagious (in spite of its name!).

Molluscum contagiosum

It is not certain how long she will be infectious but it can take anything from two to seven weeks to appear.

Home Treatment: Molluscum Contagiosum

Molluscum contagiosum usually resolves itself without treatment. But it can take up to nine months!

- **Wash your hands** after touching the lumps.

- **Use separate towels** for as long as she is infected.

- **If it itches** (it may not), soothe the skin with a bag of ice wrapped in a towel or use anti-itching medication.

- **Cantharidin** has been used since the 1950s. The cream is an extract of the blister beetle and does appear to work. But it is only used now under medical supervision and you may not find it in your pharmacy. Your doctor will apply it sparingly to any lumps, but it is not advised for the face.

- **I don't advise tape stripping** or use of irritating solutions.

- **Cryotherapy** (freezing with liquid nitrogen) can speed things up, but only if she is old enough to tolerate it.

- **No antibiotics** are needed.

- **She can go to school.**

Is It Thrush?

Many babies get nappy thrush (candidiasis) in the first three months of life. It often follows thrush in the mouth (were there white flecks inside her mouth and a white coating on her tongue that didn't scrape gently away?).

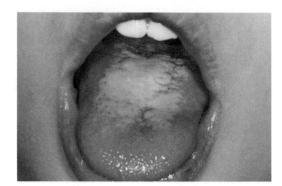

Thrush

If she has nappy thrush, you will see:

- 🧰 A nappy rash, but the skin creases around her groin will also be red.
- 🧰 The rash may spread up to the lower half of her tummy.

Thrush is more common with bottle-fed babies and they often get it after a course of antibiotics.

Home Treatment: Thrush

- ➕ Nappy thrush will respond well to **nystatin cream** (an anti-fungal antibiotic), rubbed onto the rash.
- ➕ Oral thrush responds to **nystatin gel** or to **nystatin oral suspension**.
- ➕ If it is a simple nappy rash, **barrier cream** and exposure to the **air** is best.

Is It Ringworm?

Tinea is not actually a worm – it is a fairly harmless fungal infection. Your child gets it from infected children or farm animals (not usually from your pet). The classic case is a cute, licking calf during a visit to a farm – and sucked fingers.

- 🧰 On her body, you will see red circles, with slightly raised edges.
- 🧰 On the scalp, there will be flaky patches, like dandruff. Sometimes the patch can be red and she may lose a little hair.
- 🧰 On her feet, it shows as tinea pedis – athlete's foot. You will see scaling between the toes, and broken skin.

- It is not likely to be itchy, unless she's a teenager and it's in the groin area.

- If it gets infected, she will have a big, squashy lump.

- She will spread it by direct contact. But also if she shares hairbrushes, towels, bedding or clothes.

- It's mildly infectious if left untreated.

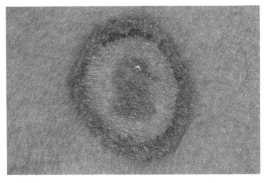

Ringworm

Home Treatment: Ringworm

- **Call your doctor** for advice about ringworm.

- **If it's body ringworm**, you can rub antifungal cream on the affected areas. Even if it clears up, make sure she continues it for four weeks.

- **If it's on the scalp**, she needs to take an oral antifungal for up to six weeks. It is much harder to shift.

- **If it's athlete's foot**, use antifungals and check her foot hygiene. Bare feet in summer works wonders.

- **No antibiotics are needed.**

- **Keep it clean** and covered with a bandage if you can.

- **Don't be tempted** to burst any swellings caused by scalp ringworm. It can cause hair loss.

- **Don't rush to the vet**; your pet is unlikely to be the cause.

- **Use separate towels** until it has cleared.

- **Put away her (cleaned) brushes and hats** for two months as the fungus hangs around.

- **Don't shave** her head or make her wear hats. It is not necessary.

- **She can go to school.**

Q&A

Q How can I know if it's just a viral infection? What will the rash look like?

A Viral infections are very common in children (the average young child gets 6–8 viral infections per year) and many will come with a rash. Often your child will have a temperature and be off form for two to three days and when the rash appears she will in fact be on the mend. There is no standard 'virus rash' but it is usually pink, it can be widespread and it always fades when you press it with your finger. The spots are usually, but not always, small. Sometimes they can be large weals: red, swollen marks. Doctors see viral rashes every day.

Q My friends overseas are surprised that we haven't vaccinated our children against the chickenpox virus. Should we?

A If it is available where you live, yes. The varicella vaccine is now widely available and it is certainly the best way to stamp out chickenpox. It has been very effective in the USA. It is expensive, though, and not every country has taken it up. Chickenpox does come with risks but these are rare and, for some countries, this vaccine is not top of the vaccine priority list. It may be easier to offer in future, with the MMRV vaccine (a combined MMR and varicella vaccine).

Remember that your child can still get chickenpox, despite a vaccine. But if she does it is likely to be mild with less fever and fewer blisters.

Q My neighbour's children have chickenpox. Should I let mine visit so they catch the virus and get it over with?

A 'Chickenpox parties' were the custom once, but I really do not subscribe to it. It is even a little reckless. Chickenpox is usually a very minor illness, but it can be serious for some children, and not only children with health problems. The problem is that you can't predict how a child will react to the virus – each has a different immune system. It is just possible that one of your children could react badly. In addition, secondary cases tend to be more severe than the first. The old way was to 'get it over with' while children were young. In fact, there is no real case for chickenpox being more serious in adults – children simply bounce back more easily.

So let's forget the chickenpox party. It is not a good idea to seek out the virus. If there is a public vaccine for chickenpox in your country, take it. If not, you could organise it privately through your doctor if you like. Anyone who has a daughter is advised to consider a blood test for antibodies when she is around twelve years old, to make sure that she has immunity for future pregnancy. (Catching the virus during pregnancy can damage the baby.) In the USA, all twelve-year-olds who test negative are vaccinated as a precaution.

Q **I've been told that she mustn't scratch the chickenpox spots, because it'll leave scars. But it's almost impossible to prevent her.**

A Scratching the spots will make the itching worse. It will not leave any marks unless the spots become infected. But they will not be permanent. When a spot gets infected, it leaves a white area of skin behind but this fades away after a few years. If it is badly infected, the skin can pucker and leave a small hole behind, but it normally heals too.

Baby Infectious Diseases

🐻 Always bring a baby with spots to the doctor. You cannot be too cautious and meningitis is a higher risk when she is small. She is most likely to get chickenpox or roseola. Her natural immunity (or lifestyle) will usually protect her from the other common infectious diseases. Chickenpox in newborns is rare but potentially very serious. They are always admitted to hospital.

Red Alert

Meningitis is always a possibility in a child with fever and a rash. Get immediate help if there are a **number of** these symptoms:

- ✚ Fever
- ✚ A flat, spotty rash that doesn't fade when pressed
- ✚ She's unusually drowsy or vomiting
- ✚ Her cry is strange
- ✚ Her hands and feet are cold
- ✚ She has a headache, stiff neck and can't tolerate bright light.

Very rarely, chickenpox can make a child seriously ill. Get help if you are concerned, especially if she is very listless or has problems breathing.

Measles, mumps, rubella and whooping cough are now rare (see Chapter 28).

Chapter 15
Nasty Parasites

'He started school in September and we've had no problems. But lately he began scratching at his head and last night I noticed something in his hair. It all got worse when I saw what was going on in there. I really don't know how I'll face his teacher.'

Itchy Heads, Bottoms and Bodies

Simply thinking about it makes some parents itch. Have 'nits' or other parasites infested the family?

I can sympathise, because there is a reasonable chance of infection if you have a school-going child. It is no cause for alarm, though. Parasites can be hard work but with a little patience you can wipe them out.

- Head lice are the most likely (but worms and scabies happen).
- None will cause any harm to your child, if treated.
- Itching is usually the first symptom.

And your child will be fascinated by them.

The days of social stigma around parasites should be well gone. After all, they did not choose one child's body because it is grubbier than the rest.

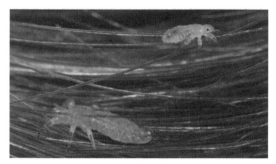

Head lice

Are They Head Lice?

Lice are the headache of every school. They usually show up when your child starts school and can be a problem until age fifteen – the 'close contact' years. Girls are most prone to them because they are serious huddlers.

Itching is usually the first thing you notice. But a lice infestation can go undetected for weeks, with **no** itching. By the time he starts to itch, there could be a decent colony of them.

- He will start complaining about itching behind his ear and the back of his neck, even his eyelashes. Then it spreads to his scalp.
- Finding a living, wriggling specimen is your best bet (if anything is alive you will soon know).

HOW BIG ARE HEAD LICE?

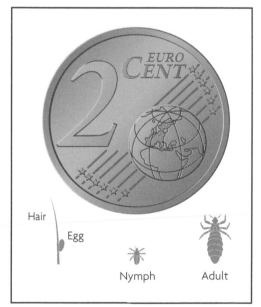

➕ What is harder is to distinguish the eggs (or egg cases) from all the usual debris in the hair – the fluff, dandruff or food. Eggs are pearly grey, oval and about the size of a pinhead. They are very like dandruff, but will not wipe off the hair as easily. They are usually at the start of hair shafts, near the scalp where it is warm, so if you find something further down the hair it is less likely to be nits.

➕ Eggs alone are not always a sign. They can stay in the scalp for weeks after the lice are dead.

The best way to test for lice is to use the Bug Busting technique (see page 178).

The Inside Track

Lice feed on human blood, so head lice spend their entire life on someone's head, apart from the odd short break on a hairbrush or hat. They are parasitic insects (pediculosis capitis), roughly the size of a sesame seed, and the female louse is the real villain. She lives on average for 30 days and can lay up to ten eggs (nits) a day. So if you do nothing about your child's lice, he will soon host a fine colony. In reality, though, an infected child will have fewer than 12 live lice on his scalp at any one time. The eggs will cling tightly to the shafts of his hair, close to the scalp where it is cosiest. It is this warmth that allows them to incubate, and the larvae emerge eight to ten days later.

Head lice do not jump. They are very opportunistic, though, and will climb quickly from hair to hair. They can also be taken by surprise. Combing hair can build up enough static electricity to physically eject an adult louse – over one metre from the host head. But travel is more usually by head-to-head contact. Household pets cannot pass them on because they do not host them; lice are only partial to human blood. They can, however, get passed on through shared hats, hair accessories, hairbrushes, rugs or pillows (an adult louse can survive up to two days without human blood).

It's the lice bites that cause the initial itching, but lice saliva and faeces worsen the irritation. So he scratches even more.

Home Treatment: Head Lice

Is he infected? If in doubt, always check the scalp within an inch of its life. No one likes insecticides, but – used with Bug Busting (see page 178) – they are still the best treatment for lice. Bug Busting alone will only work for a very committed parent.

A lice medication (chemical or physical insecticide) is the starting point.

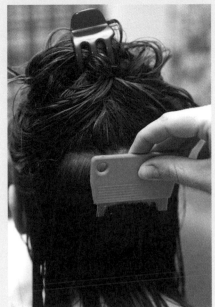

- **Wash his hair first** with a non-conditioning shampoo and towel dry it.

- **Rub the medication** into his hair, enough to wet the entire scalp. If he has long hair, it does not have to cover the ends beyond his collar.

- **Leave the ointment on** for 10 minutes and then rinse it off over the sink rather than a shower or bath (to limit exposure). The water should be cool rather than hot. Hot water dilates the scalp vessels and the less he absorbs into his scalp the better.

- **Wash the hair again** after the recommended time, to remove the ointment (use his normal shampoo).

- **'Bug bust' his hair** to remove any lice or eggs, every day or two. Insecticides are not 100 per cent effective on their own.

'Bug busting' with a lice comb will remove any lice or eggs left behind by the insecticide

- **Repeat the medication** a week later (up to 30 per cent of eggs stay alive after the first dose).

- **If you find live head lice** after dosing him, or if he gets re-infected, it is better to use a different ointment the second time. He may have a resistant strain.

- **'Bug bust' the family**, if one child is suspect. But **only** dose them if you find lice.

- **Relieve itching** (if it's bad) with an oral antihistamine.

- **Stock a bottle of lice medication** at home. You can treat his head immediately and avoid him missing school.

- **Cutting a child's hair** or tying it back does not make any difference, nor does extra shampooing or brushing. There is also no evidence that washing sheets or pillow cases matters. A scarf may be a slight barrier.

- **Have a family policy** of never sharing hairbrushes or hats.

- **He should not miss school** once he has been dosed or after the first Bug Busting session. Even if you find some nits. Alert the school, though, so other parents can check their children.

- **Never use kerosene** on a child's head.

If the treatment fails, it's nearly always because of faulty use of the medication (e.g. applying it to over-wet hair or using the wrong dosage) or because it's out of date. Or because he has been re-infected by somebody else (it happens!). Checking hair between treatments and removing any nits is very important.

Bug Busting

Bug Busting is the number one way of finding, and removing, lice and their eggs. It is simply wet combing of the hair with a special fine-toothed comb and hair conditioner.

Shampoo his hair to soak the head lice and condition it to make his hair slippery (yes, they do lose their grip!). The comb can then gently hook them out.

Comb very carefully, from the roots to the ends of the hair.

Check the hair for lice and eggs after each sweep and clear it. Wipe the comb with a white tissue or tap it onto on a white surface so you can see the contents. A magnifying glass is very useful.

Electronic combs cost more and offer no great advantage.

If you find lice or eggs, you will need to continue combing for a minimum of two weeks. Combing should be done every three days and for at least 30 minutes each time if his hair is long.

Most children actually enjoy it!

Lice Medications

➕ Permethrin (a chemical insecticide cream rubbed into the scalp) is still the most widely used. You apply it to his scalp and hair for ten minutes, after first washing and towel drying his hair.

➕ The newer dimeticone has been quite successful and appeals because it is not a chemical insecticide. It is silicone-based and it coats and smothers the lice rather than poisoning them. It works best in liquid gel form. The treatment is repeated after a week because the lotion does not seem to kill unhatched eggs. Other silicon-based treatments are available, but are not as effective.

➕ Malathion can have side effects and I only advise it where the lice seem to be resistant to permethrin. It is a chemical insecticide and comes in liquid form or lotion. It works, but the alcohol content is high, it can aggravate eczema and asthma, it is highly flammable and if it is

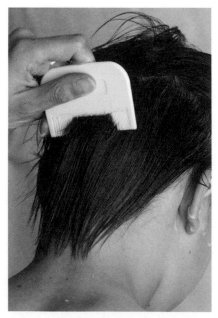

Don't stop bug busting, as medications alone are not enough

accidentally swallowed it can cause breathing problems. It is potent and only for children aged over six years.

- ⚕ Many lice treatments are not for younger children, so always check the label. I do not advise ivermectin for children as there can be side effects, especially if the treatment is not used correctly, and Lindane is no longer used in Europe.

A big problem with lice medications is the arrival of resistant strains. Permethrin, used effectively over so many years, is now facing some problems for this reason. When you use the same lotion every time, the lice eventually get used to it, especially if you under-dose them the first time. So if the lotion does not work – or your child gets a new batch of lice in school – use a different lotion next time. See if there is a pattern of resistance in your school.

Are They Worms?

These are the ones that really disturb. Especially when parents discover that their child may have worms, but show no symptoms **at all**. But before you panic – 'He's looking poorly, it must be worms' – remember that parents tend to over-diagnose them.

- ⚕ They usually cause an itchy bottom. Look for itching around the anus, especially at night. The skin around it may be peeled or red.

- ⚕ Sometimes you can see tiny worms in his stools. Or around his bottom (have a look about three hours after he falls asleep).

- ⚕ He may even (if his worm count is very high) have stomach pains and nausea.

- ⚕ The absolute test is very simple: the Sellotape test. Stick clear Sellotape onto a wooden stick, doubling it over so that the sticky side is on the outside. Press this against the skin around his anus and any eggs will stick to the tape. It is best to do the test first thing in the morning. A microscope will show them very clearly or your doctor will get it tested.

Worms do **not** cause bedwetting, teeth grinding or weight loss. And you do not get them from playing in the garden.

The Inside Track

Adult pinworms (*Enterobius vermicularis*) are like tiny white threads, roughly the length of a staple, and you can sometimes see them. Their eggs are tiny, however, and cannot be seen with the naked eye. They are also known as threadworms.

Worms first get into his body when he eats food contaminated with worm eggs. These hatch and the females busy themselves laying more eggs – on the outside skin around the anus. They actually leave the body every night to do their thing. In fact they can produce an astounding amount during their lifetime – over 10,000 eggs in three months.

His small, scratching hands can easily pick these up and when he sucks his fingers he adds to the colony inside. And so it grows.

Home Treatment: Worms

If in doubt, the Sellotape test will show if he has worms. Your doctor will confirm it.

- **Mebendazole is the best treatment.** This is an oral medicine that kills the worms. He gets a single dose, then a repeat after two weeks.
- **Some worms will survive.** Worms are hard to clear completely so try to avoid re-infection. Change his underclothes and bedclothes daily for a few weeks (if you can). Let him wear underwear under his pyjamas at night and change it every morning (for a few weeks).
- **Test the family** and any close friends. Only dose them if you find something.
- **Keep it clean.** Stop him from re-infecting by keeping his fingernails clipped, washing his hands (always before meals and after using the toilet) and giving him regular baths.
- **Keep him off school** until after the first dose of medicine. But you really must stick to the hygiene precautions.
- **You may see worms in his stools**, even after he has been treated. Don't worry – it is not unusual.

Is It Scabies?

➕ You know scabies by the itch. He won't just itch – it is so bad that he will tear at his skin. Unfortunately, it is worst at night time.

➕ He will also have a rash of little red bumps like pimples and greyish, zigzag lines where the burrows are.

➕ Where exactly he itches will depend on his age. If your child is under two, he will scratch at his head and neck, the palms of his hands and soles of his feet. If he is older, it will be in the folds of skin between his fingers, his wrists, elbows, belt line and bottom. The mites love to nestle in skin folds.

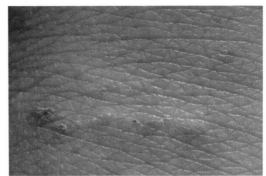

Scabies causes a rash of little red bumps and greyish, zigzag lines on the skin

In fact, the mites may have moved in a few weeks before any rash or itching starts. You can be certain it is scabies if you scrape his skin and find a mite or eggs. But they are too small to see without a microscope and we can usually diagnose it by the pattern of the rash and itching.

The Inside Track

This is not a 'dirty' problem. Scabies will infest your child if he is in contact with a carrier, no matter how well scrubbed he (or your house) is. And it's not choosy about age, sex or social background.

It is caused by a very tiny parasite that burrows under the skin and feeds on human blood. It travels through close personal contact and its droppings and eggs set up an allergic reaction, hence the itching. (If he is itching everywhere, he should also be checked out for eczema; a food allergy is less likely.)

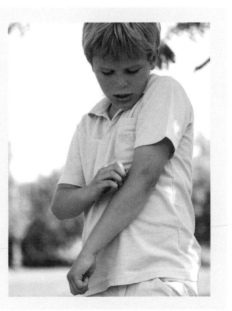

Home Treatment: Scabies

Your doctor will confirm that it is scabies.

- **An insecticide cream** will be prescribed (usually either permethrin or crotamiton, but permethrin is the drug of choice). You apply it over his entire body below his head, if he is over two years old. If he is under two years, you also have to treat the full head because scabies can affect there too.
- **Wash it off** (with a bath) after eight to 14 hours.
- **Keep him off school** until the treatment is finished.
- **Wash clothing and bed linen** he has used in the previous four days at a very high temperature.
- **Seal his toys** in plastic bags for a few weeks to kill off any strays.
- **Check the family for infection**. Only treat them if they have scabies.
- **The itching may continue**, even after the treatment has finished. It is not unusual. It may take a few weeks to die down, even though the scabies itself is gone. Oral antihistamines may help.

Treating him with medication may not be enough. He can get re-infected by bedclothes, toys or by others in your family. If he does get re-infected, the itching will start quite quickly this time.

Or Something Else?

Eczema is sometimes confused with scabies, because of the terrible itching and rash. But **where** it shows is important. Eczema usually crops up on the face, elbows, wrists and knees. If it is on his scalp and fingers too, it is likely to be scabies.

Q&A

Q I'm very reluctant to dose my child with insecticide. Surely it can't be good for him? I'd much rather use a natural remedy.

A You are right to be concerned as insecticides are toxic and some may get absorbed into the scalp. But used over a short time they are acceptable. The problems start when you pour them on indiscriminately or use them repeatedly, because no one is removing the bugs and eggs. The arrival of silicone-based insecticides is an attempt to move away from chemicals, but they are not always as effective.

In a perfect world, Bug Busting should be enough. A 2005 study in the *British Medical Journal* found that it was more effective than the standard lice medications. But it is time-consuming and needs the precision of a military operation. If you are the type of parent who can commit to serious genocide over a number of weeks, go for it. If you are the average parent with competing priorities, it is less likely to work without medication.

Tea tree oil shampoos and ointments and neem oil have become popular as an alternative way of treating lice. While products with less than 1 per cent concentration seem to be safe, it is questionable how much impact they can make. Some parents rub petroleum jelly, olive oil or mayonnaise onto the scalp, cover it with a shower cap and leave it overnight to smother the lice. Others try vinegar to dissolve the glue that attaches nits to hair. There is not a lot to show that any of this actually works (and have you ever tried getting petroleum jelly out of hair?). Bug Busting alone can be an alternative treatment for children under two years. But you need patience.

Q Can head lice cause harm?

A Head lice in themselves will do your child no harm. They are not known to transmit infectious disease and their only effect is itching, possible loss of sleep and sometimes secondary skin infection from scratching. The only harm would come from over-use of the insecticides – or misguided use of a toxic substance such as kerosene.

Baby Parasites

Babies are less likely to get infested – but they can. I always avoid using insecticides if possible. If he has head lice, you can use the Bug Busting technique alone. But with scabies, you cannot avoid using the insecticide cream. You need to cover him with cream from head to toe. With worms, I do not advise using the medication on babies under three months old.

Red Alert

If he has a rash that **does not** itch, with a fever (or seems very unwell), call your doctor. It is something else.

Chapter 16
Obesity

'She's stopped playing sports in school and I suppose I haven't pushed her, because she has a bit of asthma. Now she seems to spend all her free time in her room, at the computer or television and snacking. My family think she's put on far too much weight but what can I do? She tells me she feels breathless if she exercises.'

A Disturbing Problem

Obesity is now one of our biggest public health problems – and children have unfortunately become part of the problem. What is even more worrying, though, is the growing acceptance that to be overweight is normal. It's not. Twenty years ago, I rarely saw obese children. Now it has become alarmingly common and over a third of ten- and eleven-year-olds are either overweight or obese. That's a disturbing fact, but parents often miss the warning signs.

- Most children are obese because of their lifestyle. Only 5 per cent are genetically predisposed to it and hormones are rarely the cause.
- Obesity will damage your child's health and self-esteem, often seriously.
- Dieting is **not** the answer for an overweight child – the aim is to maintain, not lose, weight. An obese child is a different matter.

The hardest part of tackling obesity is not starting, but keeping it up. Our lifestyles work against it.

Is She Obese?

Sad to say, there is now a profile. Very typical are eight-year-olds who do not like sports and spend three hours a day in front of the computer or TV. They usually eat in front of it too, or the family eats out because of busy schedules. Their routine dinner is hamburger and fries and they are very fond of soft drinks. And they probably snore in bed at night. When tested, they will often be obese.

The international measure for obesity is the body mass index (BMI). Measuring your child's body mass on the index is a simple enough calculation. (See page 194.)

- If she measures between the 85th and 95th percentile, your child is officially overweight.*
- She is obese if her BMI is over the 95th percentile.*

The difference between being overweight and being obese is simply a matter of severity and I advise professional help in either case. Overweight children have a habit of becoming obese. Your own weight is one of the best predictors of this happening – she's ten times more likely to become obese if both parents are already obese.

* Obesity cut-offs in the US will vary.

Or Is It Something Else?

Medical causes of obesity are really very rare. Your child will not usually need tests, unless she is obese and unusually short for her age (or is under two years of age). Children who are obese from overeating are usually tall for their age.

When testing, I look for an underactive thyroid, growth hormone deficiency, Cushing's syndrome, Prader-Willi syndrome or polycystic ovarian syndrome. A child with Cushing's syndrome will be short, obese (mainly in the trunk) and have a rounded, reddened face. If she has the very rare Prader-Willi syndrome, she will be short with particularly small hands and have a voracious appetite. If she has very obvious body hair and no periods, she may have cysts on her ovaries. I always make sure that there is no depression or school problem, or an eating disorder (see page 283).

The Inside Track

When your child eats, she generates energy to power her body. In her digestive tract, the food is reduced to glucose, which is highly water soluble and can transfer easily around the body. A complex metabolic process changes this glucose into energy to keep her body cells alive and functioning. Even when resting, your child's body is burning energy (or calories). Some two-thirds of this energy is used simply to live – breathing, heart beating, etc. – and the amount she consumes for this body maintenance is her basal metabolic rate. Food processing accounts for a further 10 per cent or so of energy consumed. The rest (almost a third) of her body energy should be consumed by physical activity. If not, it is stored as fat.

The vast majority of obese children have a disturbed energy balance. The fat store never gets burned off, it simply grows. The medical world is seriously scared by obesity as the statistics keep rising. It is now a problem for developed and developing countries alike. It has even in recent years become a problem, for the first time, in sub-Saharan Africa. As income levels change, there is a change from traditional to western diets and rates of obesity rise. But it is not simply a by-product of affluence. Children from poorer areas – and females – are twice as likely to be obese as those from affluent areas.

Ironically, obesity is now seen as a form of malnutrition, with good reason. An obese child's diet lacks the nutrients that the body so badly needs.

Warning Signs

By now we have a better idea of what causes obesity. It **is** a side effect of lifestyle change.

Overeating, Especially of Energy-Dense Foods

What is your child eating? We know the ideal – food that is rich in nutrients and low in excess energy. Foods like vegetables, fruits, whole grains, pulses. The more fats, extracted sugars and refined starches in her food (the staple of most fast foods), the more energy she needs to burn off. Yet it is a sad fact that by the time children reach two years old, the most common form of vegetables they'll eat is chips. A third will eat absolutely no fruit.

And what is she drinking? Soft, carbonated drinks are insidious because she will not feel full, so she will drink more of them. If she drinks a 330 ml can every day she will move up the BMI scale by a worrying 0.18 points. But diet versions are not the answer, as the artificial sweeteners are a worry. They also keep her sweet taste buds active and that's not a good idea. She's better drinking water or fresh orange juice in sparkling water.

PORTION SIZES Have a look at the portions she eats. Everything is now double (or even treble) the size it was some twenty years ago – fast food servings, chocolate bars, lunch rolls. She is probably eating twice what you ate at the same age. A large fast food meal could contain 2,200 kcal, which would take a full marathon race to burn off. If she is a child, she should eat a child's portion – not an adult's.

CHILD-SIZED PORTIONS

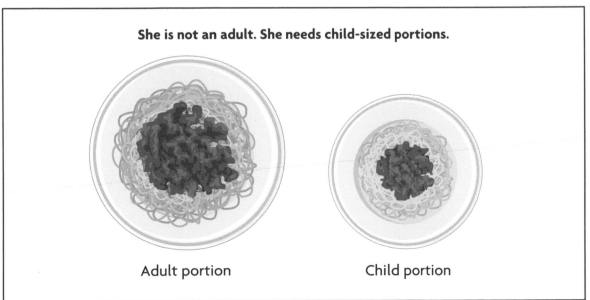

She is not an adult. She needs child-sized portions.

Adult portion   Child portion

PORTION SIZES

Twenty years ago		Today
1 portion = 500 calories	Spaghetti and meatballs	1 portion = 1,025 calories
85 calories	Soft drink	250 calories (35 minutes' exercise to burn off)
210 calories	French fries	610 calories (1 hour 10 minutes' walking to burn off)
333 calories	Hamburger	590 calories
55 calories	Cookie	275 calories

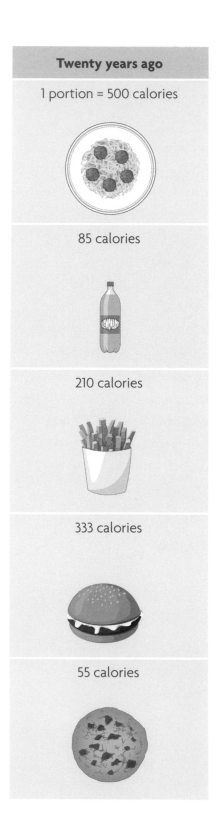
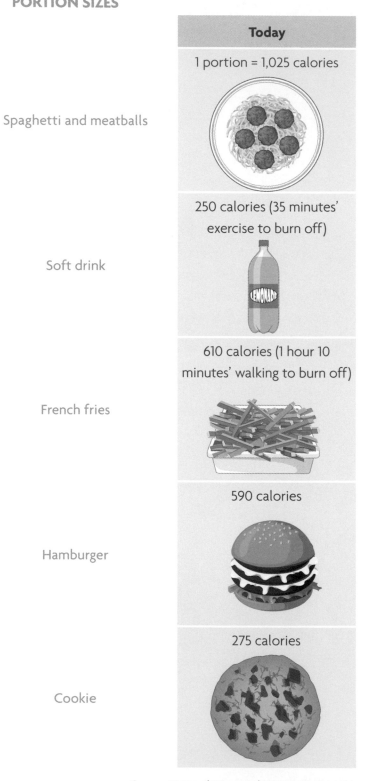

Source: National Heart and Lung Institute, USA.

Too Much Computer and Television Time

How much screen time does she have? It is one of the biggest causes of obesity because it keeps children inactive for long periods – and because they passively eat energy-dense snacks. Your five-year-old's chances of being an obese adult rise by 8 per cent for every extra hour of television she watches a day. And having a television in her room makes it worse. The National Health and Nutrition Survey in the USA found that it was a strong predictor of being overweight.

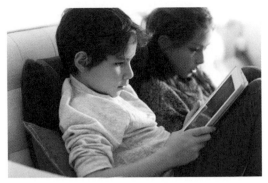

Too much screen time is one of the biggest causes of childhood obesity

Family Lifestyles: Eating out or Takeaways

How often do you have family meals? Hectic schedules mean that families are eating together – at home – less often. Many are spending half their weekly food budget on eating out or on takeaway food. Skipping breakfast, snacking and eating out have all been associated with obesity. If she has scheduled family meals, she is less likely to eat junk food, portions can be controlled and she is more likely to eat less because she eats more slowly and snacks less often.

A Progressive Decline in Exercise

How much exercise is she getting every day? What chance has she of burning everything off? Safety in school yards and busy school curricula mean that children may have less scheduled exercise time than before. And adolescents often drop out of organised sport as it becomes more competitive.

Large Food Marketing Budgets

Our children's eating habits are not helped by heavy and high-profile marketing by the fast food industry. There has been pressure to ban the advertising of junk food for children. Now there is also pressure to address the food and drink itself, and some countries (Denmark and France) have even introduced fat and sugar taxes. The fast food industry is beginning to react, but very slowly. The very unsafe trans fats (partially hydrogenated oil) in fast food are likely to be phased out or banned, but they may still appear in some shops. Look for 'partially hydrogenated oils' in the ingredients list of any packet of processed food and avoid it. Better still, avoid processed food! A number of fast food companies have now removed soft drinks from their menus, but governments may take more drastic action on health grounds.

The Damage Obesity Causes

Children are now showing medical conditions that were previously exclusive to adults. Most worrying is the fact that nearly half of all severely obese children now have Type 2 diabetes.

If your child is obese, she is creating serious problems for herself:

- Type 2 diabetes.
- Asthma.
- High cholesterol and hypertension leading to heart disease.
- Sleep apnoea.
- Gallstones.
- Liver disease.
- Joint problems and, in the long term, osteoarthritis.
- Puberty and menstrual problems.
- Clinical depression.

Obesity is likely to take over from smoking as the leading cause of death. It has already been flagged as a leading cause of cancer in the future.

But the psychological effects of obesity can also be devastating. Your child will be vulnerable to bullying and isolation from her own age group, and obesity has been shown to influence careers; studies are now showing clear signs of obesity discrimination. If she stays obese, her chances of being selected for a job and her starting salary are likely to be affected when she is older.

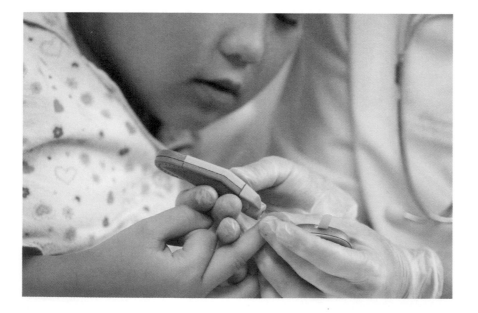

Blood sugar measurement being taken in a young diabetic child. Obesity creates serious health problems, including Type 2 diabetes.

No Diets, No Surgery

It will take some drastic social changes to make a real dent in obesity: tighter controls on food advertising and on the quality of our food and drink; better urban planning to get people out of their cars; easy and cheap access to fresh foods. All you can do is change things in your own family.

Putting your overweight child on a diet is **not** the answer. Rigid diets are harmful to their growing bodies and doctors will only consider a diet in exceptional cases. In fact (and this important for children who are overweight), forget about losing weight. Your aim is to keep her at the **same** weight – so that she slims naturally as she grows. It is only if she is obese that some weight will need to be (slowly) lost.

Your best move is to consider your family lifestyle, the likely root of her problem. Then introduce small, but incremental, changes in eating and exercise habits. And make sure you have professional support.

Drug treatment for obesity is never advised for a child under twelve years of age. Even with adolescents, it should only be prescribed where there are medical complications or where the obesity is causing serious psychological problems. As for bariatric surgery (basically decreasing the stomach size by stapling), this should only be considered for children and adolescents in rare cases, as a last resort: if the BMI is over 40 or if there is a serious medical complication and all other efforts have failed.

Home Treatment: Weight Problems

If your child has a weight problem, your best move will be finding a determined doctor or dietician to help.

Treating her weight problem will only work if it is a family decision and you all subscribe to it. At her age, the biggest change will come from exercise.

If she is overweight (but not obese):

- **Don't put her on a diet.** It won't work long term and rapid weight loss can be harmful to growing children. Only adolescents who have stopped growing can safely lose around 0.5 kg a week. Your best chance of success in changing food habits is to change the habits of the whole family and to seek help from a dietician or nutritionist.
- **Make sure that she gets enough sleep.** The less children sleep, the more likely they are to be obese.
- **Exercise trade-offs** Even one extra hour's exercise a week can noticeably reduce her BMI.

- **The recommended minimum** for children is 30 minutes' exercise a day, and ideally 60 minutes for a school-going child.

  - For a toddler, pottering around the house or garden will be enough.

  - Start with simple changes and get the whole family exercising. Run up the stairs; walk rather than drive whenever you can. Try a ten-minute walk together before bed. Or a family cycle at the weekend.

  - Be creative in winter. How can she exercise indoors? Try exercise DVDs, playroom aerobics, a trampoline, or bundle her up for a walk in the rain.

  - Trade exercise for screen time. Every half hour of activity buys her a half hour of TV or computer.

  - Agree a daily quota of screen time (up to the recommended maximum of two hours daily), but let her decide how she uses it.

  - Don't keep a TV or computer in her bedroom.

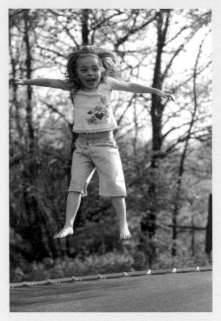

Increasing the amount of exercise your child takes is much better than putting her on a diet

- **Less energy-dense food.** It is useful to keep a 'food diary' for a few weeks to see how much of your family food and drink is high in calories but low on nutrition. Encourage her to help you.

- **Agree healthy meal menus** that she can live with instead, and involve her in cooking where you can. Do not fall into the trap of offering biscuits and sweets as rewards, or to comfort her. Attention and hugs are the best comfort.

- Very importantly, **get her portion sizes right**. Agree standard portions for her cereals, meat and other standard foods, using her hand or a measuring jug to size them. She is a child, so she should eat a child's portion.

- **More fresh food.** The best foods are whole foods that take time to eat, such as fruits or wholemeal bread. Let her eat as much fruit and vegetables as she likes, ideally at least five portions a day. If she 'hates vegetables', keep trying tiny tastes and she will – eventually! – accept them. Try soups, fun fruit plates, fruit salads with her favourite ice cream, food games, anything that will entice her. (It is much easier if you start when she is small.) Smoothies are good, but not if they have too much banana; and don't overdo them as they are not as good as fresh, unsqueezed fruit (make sure they are not sweetened). If weekday cooking cannot be scheduled, can you make a pot of food at the weekend and freeze it? And can you part with your frying pan?

- **Substitute foods** Agree substitutes for one energy-dense food at a time. Maybe dried fruits for processed snacks, corn on the cob for waffles, home-made chicken wraps for sausage rolls. Start substituting drinks too, and move her away from soft, carbonated drinks to milk, pure juice and – best of all – water. (It's useful to bring a water bottle everywhere in the car.) Low-fat milk is a good idea once she is over two years old, but not before.

- ⊞ **Don't give your child soft drinks**, energy drinks or flavoured mineral waters.

- ⊞ **Family mealtimes.** One surprisingly effective move is to bring back family meals. Even one shared meal a day will make a difference. Make sure that:

  - ✛ Meals happen in the kitchen.
  - ✛ Meals are scheduled and last 20 to 30 minutes.
  - ✛ TV, radio and mobile phones are turned off.
  - ✛ **You** serve the food to control the portions.

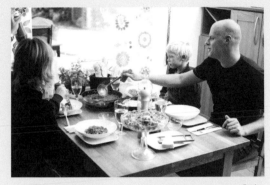

- ⊞ **Watch her self-esteem** Give her specific techniques to cope with teasing and make sure there is no underlying emotional issue. Praise every success, no matter how small, and keep very positive.

Family mealtimes are a great way to fight obesity

- ⊞ **Pace yourself.** Don't start a food and exercise revolution. But do start this month and let everyone in the family know why it is important.

- ⊞ **Start with you.** You are her champion; she will copy you.

- ⊞ All children older than two years should have their **BMI checked** at least annually. If she's already overweight or obese, it should be checked every three months.

- ⊞ If she is obese, she will need **medical support** as a matter of urgency.

Body Mass Index Charts

The body mass index (BMI) is our most practical measure of obesity. The charts on the following pages show the cut-offs for obesity and overweight in children, as recommended by the International Obesity Task Force. (You need to be a little careful in interpreting them, especially as your child's BMI can change during normal growth.) Talk to your doctor if your child's BMI is in the unhealthy areas.

Measuring your child's body mass on the index is a simple enough calculation. Take her height, multiply it by the same figure – then divide her weight by the result.

$$BMI = \frac{\text{weight in kilograms}}{\text{height in metres (squared)}}$$

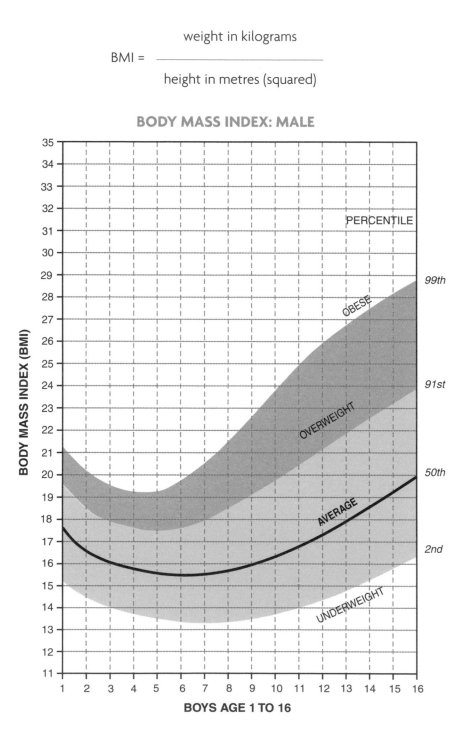

BODY MASS INDEX: MALE

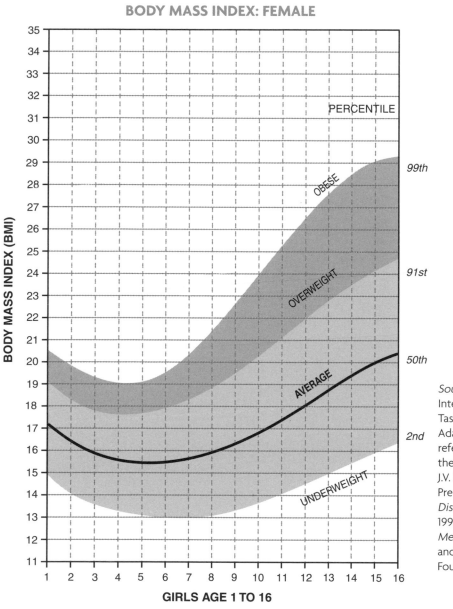

BODY MASS INDEX: FEMALE

GIRLS AGE 1 TO 16

Sources: Based on International Obesity Task Force BMI charts. Adapted from the BMI reference curve for the UK, 1990 (T.J. Cole, J.V. Freeman and M.A. Preece) *Archives of Disease in Childhood* 1995, 73: 25–9; *British Medical Journal* 2000 and Child Growth Foundation; *BMJ* 2007.

Q&A

Q She's only seven and still developing. The doctor says she's overweight, but I think she'll grow out of it. It looks like puppy fat to me.

A Look long and hard at her lifestyle and eating habits – then trust your instincts. If you're happy that she's eating and exercising enough, you may be right. Her BMI should bear this out. She may lose the fat as she grows, but I would not depend on it. At puberty, most boys lose some body fat but 30 per cent of obese boys don't. Unfortunately, body fat tends to increase in girls at this stage.

Q Are some children simply more prone to getting fat?

A The biggest impact on a child's body weight is their food and activity habits. Even small changes in these habits can affect weight quite strikingly. If she eats an extra one hundred calories a day (just two chocolates) she will gain an extra pound a month. Unless she burns it off.

It need not be overly strenuous to be effective:

✚ 45 minutes of dancing burns some 450 calories.

✚ 90 minutes of football burns some 600 calories.

There is a belief that obese children usually have a slow metabolism. This a myth.

A very small percentage of children will use less energy so they will be more prone to becoming overweight or obese. With this 5 per cent group, genetics can influence the rate at which they use energy. But lifestyle will ultimately make them fat or slim. Sometimes poor nutrition in early childhood (or before birth) can affect the way a body uses energy – ironically, it may increase the chances of obesity. Bottle-fed children also seem to be at a higher risk of obesity. In 2015, the World Commission on Ending Childhood Obesity recommended breastfeeding a child for the first six months, for this reason.

Q How much exercise does a school-going child need?

A The recommended amount is now 60 minutes a day, but it does not have to be organised sports. It can be enough to play in the garden with friends or to run about in the school yard. A half-hour of unstructured free play will help to burn up a toddler's calories. What is important is to get children off the sofa and moving.

Any increase in physical activity will help. Your child has little real control over her basal metabolic rate, but she has considerable control over the amount of energy she burns through exercise.

Q I don't want to put my child on a diet, but I do want to give her some guidelines about eating. What do you suggest?

A The Traffic Light or 'Go, Slow and Whoa' diet is used for children aged six to twelve years old and is worth trying. It offers her three types of food: green foods, such as fruit and vegetables, are low-energy and high-nutrient; orange foods are moderate-energy; and red foods are high-energy. She can eat 'green' foods often, 'orange' foods in moderation and 'red' foods sparingly.

THE TRAFFIC LIGHT DIET

FOOD GROUP	GO (almost any time foods)	SLOW (sometimes foods)	WHOA (once in a while foods)
	Nutrient dense ⟵	⟶	Calorie-dense
Vegetables	Almost all fresh, frozen and canned vegetables without added fat and sauces	All vegetables with added fat and sauces; oven-baked French fries; avocado	Fried potatoes, like French fires and hash browns; other deep-fried vegetables
Fruits	All fresh, frozen and canned in juice	100 per cent fruit juice; fruits canned in light syrup; dried fruits	Fruits canned in heavy syrup
Breads and cereals	Wholegrain breads, including pita bread; tortillas and wholegrain pasta; brown rice; hot and cold unsweetened wholegrain breakfast cereals	White refined flour bread, rice and pasta; French toast; taco shells; cornbread; biscuits; granola; waffles and pancakes	Croissants; muffins; doughnuts; sweet rolls; crackers made with trans fats; sweetened breakfast cereals
Milk and milk products	Fat-free or 1 per cent low-fat milk; fat-free or low-fat yoghurt; part-skin, reduced fat and fat-free cheese; low-fat and fat-free cottage cheese	2 per cent low-fat milk; processed cheese spread	Whole milk; full-fat American, cheddar, Colby, Swiss and cream cheese; whole-milk yoghurt
Meats, poultry, fish, eggs, beans and nuts	Trimmed beef and pork; extra lean ground beef; chicken and turkey without skin; tuna canned in water; baked, broiled, steamed and grilled fish and shellfish; beans, split peas, lentils and tofu; egg whites and egg substitutes	Lean ground beef and broiled hamburgers; ham and Canadian bacon; chicken and turkey with skin; low-fat hot dogs; tuna canned in oil; peanut butter; nuts; whole eggs cooked without added fat	Untrimmed beef and pork; regular ground beef; fried hamburgers; ribs; bacon; friend chicken and chicken nuggets; hot dogs, lunch meats, pepperoni and sausage; fried fish and shellfish; whole eggs cooked with fat
Sweets and snacks		Ice milk bars; frozen fruit juice bars; low-fat or fat-free frozen yoghurt and ice cream; fig bars; ginger snaps; backed chips; low-fat microwave popcorn; pretzels	Cookies and cakes; pies; cheesecake; ice cream; chocolate; candy; chips; buttered microwave popcorn
Fats/condiments	Vinegar; ketchup; mustard; fat-free creamy salad dressing; fat-free mayonnaise; fat-free sour cream	Vegetable oil, olive oil and oil-based salad dressing; soft margarine; low-fat creamy salad dressing; low-fat mayonnaise; low-fat sour cream	Butter and stick margarine; lard; salt pork; gravy; regular creamy salad dressing; mayonnaise; tartar sauce; sour cream; cheese sauce; cream sauce; cream cheese dips
Beverages	Water; fat-free milk and 1 per cent low-fat milk; diet soda; unsweetened iced tea and diet iced tea; lemonade	2 per cent low-fat milk; 100 per cent fruit juice; sports drinks	Whole milk; regular soda; calorifically sweetened iced teas and lemonade; fruit drinks with less than 100 per cent fruit juice

Source: National, Heart, Lung and Blood Institute, USA. Adapted from *CATCH: Coordinated Approach to Child Health*, 4th Grade Curriculum, University of California and Flaghouse, Inc., 2002.

Baby Obesity

🐻 If you have the choice, breastfeed. It lowers your child's chances of becoming obese later by up to 25 per cent. The longer she's breastfed, the less likely she is to become obese.

🐻 Always follow the instructions when preparing formula milk. Don't be tempted to add a little extra. And don't give her extra bottles just because she's crying. Let her suck on a small water bottle instead. Try not to give her fruit juices or biscuits for snacks. Get her used to water and fruit snacks.

🐻 Let her crawl free as much as possible. Don't leave her for long periods in a baby seat or buggy.

Red Alert

TALK TO YOUR DOCTOR:

➕ If you have any concerns about her weight.

➕ If you believe that your child is obese.

➕ Before starting any weight treatment.

➕ If she is obese and unusually short for her age, or under two years. She may need further tests for a medical condition.

➕ If she seems to have depression problems.

Your child will be referred to a specialist if obesity has caused sleep apnoea, hypertension, orthopaedic problems or Type 2 diabetes (also if she is 'super obese' with a BMI somewhere around 40). Only children who have severe health risks from obesity need to lose weight quickly – and always under the care of an obesity centre. Drug treatment and surgery for obesity are not suitable for children.

If she is depressed as well as obese, she really needs a psychologist to work alongside her. Treating her weight alone will not be enough.

Chapter 17

Penis & Foreskin Problems

'He's acting up when I try to get him to do a wee, even though I know he needs to. The tip of his penis has become raw red and I think it may be hurting when he goes.'

Sensitive Areas

It is not just zippers that cause penis problems. Your boy will almost certainly have some problem with his penis before his teens. It can be a sensitive area in more ways than one, especially when a parent is squeamish. But most of what crops up is very normal. After all:

- 🔒 60 per cent of boys have foreskin 'problems' at one to two years of age. But they usually self-correct.
- 🔒 Inflammation is very common and easily treated.
- 🔒 Circumcision is rarely advised for penis problems.
- 🔒 Zipper injuries are more common than you think.

BUT

Any pain or swelling should always be checked out.

Is It a Penis Problem?

FORESKIN ATTACHED is usually the first concern for parents. The foreskin protects the sensitive tip of the penis (glans) with its loose hood of skin. A common worry is when parents notice that the foreskin is attached to the tip. But nearly all boys are born with the foreskin attached (non-retractile). It is normal and even at one year 60 per cent of foreskins will be attached in some way. By four years old 90 per cent have finally separated and the rest will part ways by puberty.

INFLAMMATION happens a lot and for any number of reasons. Something has caused irritation – perhaps soaps, bath oils or simply wet nappies. Or have you been trying to work his foreskin back too vigorously?

- 🔒 Is the tip of his foreskin a little red?
- 🔒 Is it sore?

BALANITIS The penis is usually badly inflamed, because of an infection:

- 🔒 Is the tip of his penis and foreskin **very** red and sore?
- 🔒 There may be pus at the end of the foreskin.
- 🔒 The penis opening may have narrowed.
- 🔒 His penis may even be very swollen.

SMEGMA is sometimes wrongly diagnosed as a cyst, especially when it produces a sizeable swelling – as it can.

+ Are there small yellow or white lumps under his foreskin?

+ Can you feel them or even see them?

If so, it is likely to be smegma and perfectly harmless, especially if he is under four. This is because his foreskin may still be attached to the penis. When his skin secretes oils, they can get clogged under the foreskin and cause small lumps.

PHIMOSIS The tip of the foreskin is so tightly narrowed that it cannot be pulled back:

+ You cannot see the opening at the tip of his penis.

+ When he urinates, the foreskin 'balloons'.

+ The foreskin opening is as small as a pinhole.

+ When he urinates, the stream is very narrow.

FORESKIN PROBLEMS

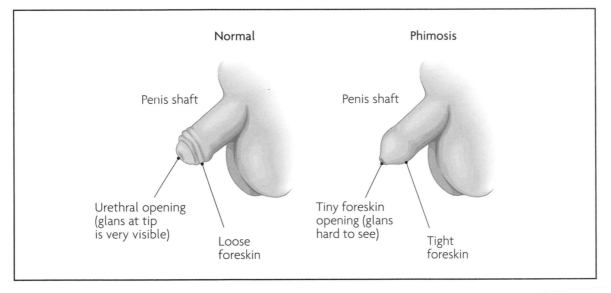

Normal

Penis shaft

Urethral opening
(glans at tip
is very visible)

Loose
foreskin

Phimosis

Penis shaft

Tiny foreskin
opening (glans
hard to see)

Tight
foreskin

OTHER PENIS PROBLEMS

Hair tourniquet	You may find that something has wrapped itself round his penis and is pulled tight – often a tiny thread from his clothes or a tiny hair. Is the base of the penis (near his crotch) red and swollen? Can you see a fine line?
Zipper injury	It happens. But they learn fast. Did he get his foreskin caught in the zip of his trousers?
Paraphimosis	Sometimes the foreskin is left pulled back and becomes quite swollen. Is his foreskin so swollen that it's hard to pull forward? Is it painful?
Hypospadias	There are two problems here and it is usually picked up at birth. First, the opening of the urethra is not at the tip of his penis as it should be – it is under the tip. And second, the penis is bent forward slightly. Does his foreskin look almost square? Is it hanging off his penis?

Or Something Else?

Sometimes the penis is not actually the problem.

If it hurts or burns him when he urinates, he may have a urinary tract infection. Swelling in the scrotum can be caused by a hydrocoele, which is best left alone. Swelling in the groin is usually an inguinal hernia.

Undescended testes (they don't come down!) are another matter. The problem is generally picked up at birth and it is not unusual: 1 in 20 boys are born with it. Usually they descend naturally and by one year only 1 in 50 baby boys will still have a problem and need a simple operation called an orchidopexy. Ideally he will have the operation before his first birthday. Sometimes it may be picked up later and it's important to correct it as it can affect his fertility.

Incidentally, boys have a great ability to pull back their testes. Many apparently undescended testes are in fact retractile; they shoot up into the groin when cold hands touch the scrotum.

The Inside Track

In all bodies, the sex organs are linked to the urinary system – which is why it is known as the urogenital system. In your boy, everything converges on the penis and especially the urethra: the internal tube through which urine and semen have to pass on their way out of the body. The urethra runs from his bladder, up the penis shaft to the urethral opening at the tip of his penis. This tip is the 'glans', which is full of nerve endings and a very sensitive area – as he will learn early enough. It is a distinct structure covered by the protective foreskin (a double layer of skin, which is very mobile). It is also very sensitive to any impact or swelling and can get very swollen quickly, even from a relatively small insect bite. The blood supply to the glans is a separate system from the rest of the penis.

BOYS' URINARY SYSTEM

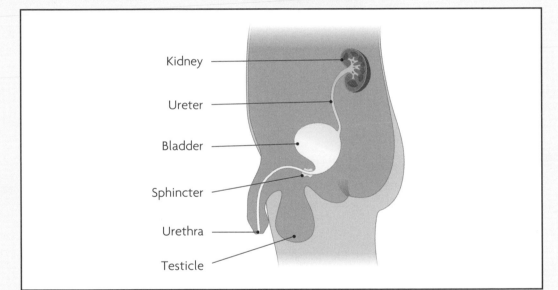

Kidney

Ureter

Bladder

Sphincter

Urethra

Testicle

The penis itself is mainly spongy tissue (capable of filling with blood to become erect) and has no bones or muscles in it. Inside, there are three spongy tubes, one of which carries the urethra. Despite all the schoolboy jokes, the size of his penis has nothing to do with how well it works.

The penis is cased in a thick membrane so that when it fills with blood it is a firm structure. In fact, the whole structure of the penis is tougher than it seems, so it can take quite a lot of impact.

Home Treatment: Penis & Foreskin Problems

Once your child's foreskin is moving freely, get him in the habit of pulling it back gently when he is showering or bathing. It will keep everything healthy. **Never force** his foreskin back. It could over-tighten and his penis could get damaged. But if you have forced it and it now will not move forward, contact your doctor at once. Some penis problems you can handle yourself, others will need help.

- **Foreskin attached.** It usually sorts itself out, and eventually his foreskin will pull back. No one needs to get involved – unless the penis is badly inflamed or swollen. Or unless he is four years old and the foreskin is still not moving.

- **Minor inflammation.** Any good nappy barrier cream will do the trick. Along with tackling whatever caused the irritation. But if it gets very sore and swells or the opening narrows, bring him to the doctor.

- **Balanitis.** See your doctor. A steroid cream (1 per cent hydrocortisone on prescription) can help. So will soaking in a warm (not hot) bath – ideally with the foreskin very gently pulled back. If it is severe, he may need antibiotics.

- **Smegma.** You do not have to do anything. Smegma always works its own way out. It may be a little sore and red for a few days afterwards but this is normal.

- **Zipper injury.** Do not try to free him yourself; bring him to the doctor or hospital at once. Try numbing the area a little with ice in the meantime. Freeing him is going to be very painful so he will need painkillers, and maybe a sedative, before anyone tries. He will also get a generous dose of anaesthetic cream on the trapped area. Then the zipper can be eased down gently or cut.

- **Hair tourniquet.** Work the thread or hair loose very gently. Do not try cutting it in a panic! If you cannot loosen it, bring him to your doctor at once. Even if you do manage to release him, get him checked out for any injury.

- **Phimosis.** See your doctor. It may simply be a foreskin that has not separated yet. But if it is phimosis, he will be prescribed a steroid cream for a month, which usually cures the problem completely. The steroid makes the skin thinner and looser for a short time so that it can be pulled back. It also brings the inflammation down. He will only need circumcision if the steroids do not work.

- **Paraphimosis.** Bring him to the hospital at once, where they can usually solve the problem by gently manipulating his foreskin so that it moves forward, and by gently squeezing any fluid out. Sometimes covering the area with a large dollop of anaesthetic cream is enough. But it is very painful and he will need to be very patient so they will probably give him painkillers or, if it is severe, sedation. If they cannot do it manually, he will need surgery and if it happens again, he may need circumcision.

- ✚ **Hypospadias.** See your doctor. Your child will need surgery to right everything and the results are usually excellent. He will not (and should not) be circumcised, as he will need the foreskin to repair hypospadias.

Q&A

Q His foreskin has become inflamed again and I'm wondering if circumcision is on the cards.

A Circumcision is the surgical removal of the foreskin from the penis. There is a good deal of debate about circumcision and some religious groups insist on it. But it is rarely advised today on medical grounds and most international paediatric bodies do not recommend circumcision as routine. There are a few exceptions, such as a child with severe phimosis who does not respond to steroids. It's a treatment of last resort, if all other treatments fail to work.

There are arguments that circumcised children may have less risk of urinary tract infections. But the evidence is not fully convincing and the problems circumcision can cause will outweigh any benefits. Problems include bleeding and infection; inflammation of the glans penis; and the fact that, of course, circumcision hurts like hell and can be traumatic for a child. With good hygiene practices, an uncircumcised penis will be as clean as a circumcised one. It is a significant operation and, in my book, a child has to 'earn' circumcision.

Q My teenage son has a very sore testicle – what should I do?

A He needs to see your doctor right away and the worry here is that he may have a torsion (twist) of the testis. This will give him symptoms such as pain in the testicle, and the testicle itself may feel hard and lie higher than on the other side. He may also feel sick and have stomach pains. If torsion is suspected, he will be referred to hospital urgently and an ultrasound will check it out. But if the test rules out torsion, then he very likely has orchitis. This is usually caused by a virus and makes the testicle very painful, tender and swollen.

Baby Penis Problems

🐻 The most common genital problem in baby boys is hypospadias, but it is usually spotted at birth.

🐻 Hydroceles (too much fluid around the testes) is very common in newborns and will resolve itself. He will not need any treatment.

Red Alert

CONTACT YOUR DOCTOR IMMEDIATELY IF:

✚ There is any swelling or pain in the penis. Or if he has trouble passing urine.

✚ There is reddened swelling in his groin that's tender to touch and you cannot push it back. It may be a strangulated hernia.

✚ His testes are sore, swollen and tender. It's most likely orchitis, an infection. But if it's torsion, he needs urgent help.

Chapter 18

Recurring Headaches & Tummy Pains

'She's eleven, and over the past three months she's started to have these headaches. Maybe two or three times a week and they're always quite bad. She's missed about six days of school by now, which is a pity because she's doing really well. She's always top of the class and into everything that's going: gymnastics, dance, guitar. Her aunt had a brain haemorrhage last year and we're very worried.'

Children Do Get Headaches

It is not just an adult thing – most school-age children have had headaches. It's worrying, however, if your child seems to get them often. Is something more ominous going on? Probably not.

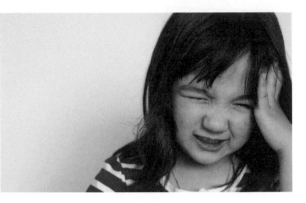

- Most recurring headaches are caused by tension – or migraine.
- A short history of headaches that worsen by the week is a concern.
- Less worrying are headaches that have not changed over 12 months.
- A clear picture of the headache pattern is really important.

Time and again, parents push for CT or MRI scanning – 'just in case' – but a medical examination will rule out anything serious. Scans are usually not needed and will expose her to a sizeable amount of radiation.

Headaches are rarely serious, but always bring a child with recurring headaches to see your doctor.

BUT

If the headache comes with other symptoms, or is worsening, call your doctor at once.

Is It Migraine?

It is not quite the same as adult migraine, but it can floor them just as much. Migraine can start as young as five and it affects about one in nine children under the age of fifteen. It's probably migraine if:

- It is a throbbing headache.
- It is severe and seems to bore into the back of her eyes.
- It lasts more than an hour or two.
- Her face is ghostly pale.
- She just wants to curl up and do nothing.

Sometimes the effects can be quite frightening. Your child may feel dizzy, have temporary loss of vision or slur her speech. She may even lose power on one side of her body for a short time.

It's almost certainly migraine if she has other symptoms too:

- She feels sick or vomits.
- She shies away from light or loud noises.
- There is a family history of headaches.
- She wants to sleep.

If it is a bad migraine, it can appear quite quickly. She will drop her toys and sneak away to a dark corner or room, lie down and fall asleep. The headache will usually be gone when she wakes up. If she still has a headache on Day Two, it is less likely to be migraine.

Will she grow out of it? Some do, but it may stay, especially if your child is female, if the headaches started before the age of six and if there is a family history of migraine (headaches tend to run in families, especially migraine). If it is any consolation, it will ease off, but it may be as late as middle age. Remember that, painful as it is, there is no serious problem with her brain.

Migraine Triggers

She will have her own triggers, which might include:

- Stress.
- Lack of food.
- Not drinking enough fluids.
- Extreme activity, such as competitive sports.
- Some foods.
- Puberty with its hormone changes.

It is most often caused by stress (or, if the girl has reached puberty, by the rush of oestrogen just before menstruation).

THE COMMON CAUSES OF MIGRAINE HEADACHES IN CHILDREN

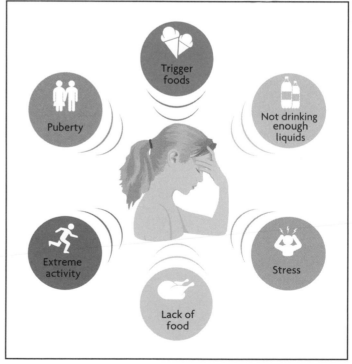

Is It a Tension Headache?

It is a bit disconcerting to be told that your child is stressed. But tension headaches are not unusual for children. On the positive side, this type of headache is the most likely to disappear with time – and a little help. The headache will usually have these symptoms:

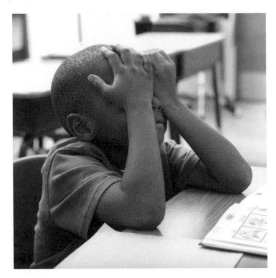

- ⊞ It is unlikely to throb.
- ⊞ It is frequent and can last 30 minutes or several days.
- ⊞ Her neck will be tense.
- ⊞ The pain will be manageable, rather than severe.
- ⊞ The pain will be in her forehead or like a tight band around her head.
- ⊞ It is unlikely to cause vomiting.

She will be able to go about her daily business but she will not be a happy camper. Worrying about the headaches will make it all worse.

These are sometimes called 'psychosomatic headaches', which is unfair to any child who is feeling real pain. Very often, tension headaches can be traced to a school problem such as bullying or an overdose of after-school activities. Do they go away – strangely – at weekends or during holidays? Is she good at everything but spun out by too much homework or too many hobbies? Recent studies have shown that these headaches happen most often during the first 12 months of starting school. But they can also be triggered by home tensions or a major family event such as a death or moving home. She may get a crop of headaches just before puberty, when everything is happening in her life. Look at her weekly routine and all the possible stressors in her life.

Or Something Else?

Most children with a serious headache who end up in hospital have an infection, either viral or respiratory. It is usually a one-off headache and it soon disappears. Where headaches recur, this is normally because of migraine or tension. More rarely, there can be another cause.

BRAIN TUMOUR It is your worst fear, but a brain tumour is really very rare (3 in every 100,000 children). It is not, in fact, the tumour that causes headaches but raised pressure on the base of the brain from a build-up of fluid.

If it's a tumour, there will be other symptoms apart from the headaches:

➕ Her movements may puzzle you: Why is she confused, unsteady on her feet?

➕ Why does she tilt her head?

➕ Why is her speech slurred?

➕ Her personality may also seem to change: has she become very difficult, are there sudden rages?

The headaches will be felt anywhere in the head. What is most telling is:

➕ A headache that wakes her and is worst in the morning, improving during the day and which eases off if she vomits.

➕ A story of mild headaches that have risen quickly to a crescendo of severe and frequent headaches.

Headaches that are frequent, but unchanged, over 12 months are unlikely to mean a brain tumour.

BENIGN INTRACRANIAL HYPERTENSION is quite rare and is not serious. Pressure within the brain is raised, often for no clear reason, but certainly not because of any obstruction. Drugs can be a cause, especially overuse of vitamin A. But the symptoms are similar to a brain tumour and (if she has them) she will need a scan to rule out a tumour.

SINUSITIS If she has sinusitis, her headache will be dull and throbbing and she will feel it around the cheekbones under her eyes – not on the forehead. It may get worse if she coughs or bends over.

SHUNT BLOCKAGE If she has hydrocephalus (and a shunt was inserted) I always check for shunt problems.

EYE STRAIN is not, as often believed, a common cause of headaches. But vision should always be checked.

The Inside Track

Parents often see pain as a sign of a serious problem. They feel that something must be wrong simply because pains have lasted so long. In fact, the reverse is true. The shorter the duration, the more likely it is that the pain is due to something serious. Pain is very personal, so it can be hard to pin down a child's headache. A dull pain to one can be sharp to another. Of course, a two-year-old feels pain, but how can she describe it? She may simply cry or rock, hide in a corner or act up. If the pain is chronic, she may go off her food and have problems sleeping. It is more useful to look at the pattern of her headaches – where it is sore and when it happens.

What is making her head ache? With migraine, there is a spasm of the blood vessels in her head and neck, causing a temporary drop in the flow of blood. Her brain compensates by increasing the blood flow and the extra pressure on the area produces a throbbing, migraine headache. Many people experience an 'aura' (flashing lights or strange sensations) when the spasm starts and it can be an early warning signal. Migraine tends to run in families.

The Headache Pattern

Doctors need to know the pattern of the headaches. I always advise parents to start a headache diary to find out:

How long?
When did they start, and have they become more frequent or more severe?

What's a headache episode like?
Describe how the headache feels, where it is, how long it lasts and if there are any other symptoms.

Timing
Do headaches tend to happen in the evening or early morning, just on schooldays or at weekends and holidays too?

Triggers
Does anything seem to trigger the headaches? Have there been any major family changes?

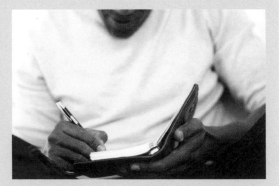

Keeping a headache diary is a good way to track your child's headache patterns

Her reaction

What does your child do to relieve the headache? Lie down? Is she quick to take a painkiller?

School days lost

This is important as it may point to a school problem.

Remedies tried

Painkillers, changes in diet, home remedies and anything you have tried to prevent the headaches.

Family history

It is important to know if migraine is in the family but also if there is any history of brain haemorrhage or tumour.

Home Treatment: Headaches

With a recurring headache, she needs a full neurological examination and your doctor can do this in the surgery. Everything will be checked: full cranial nerve and eye examination, head size, height and weight centiles, blood pressure, pulse rate, skin (for unusual signs), vision, signs of a head tilt, how she walks and limb tendon reflexes. You should also keep a 'headache diary' at home to see the pattern of headaches. Once anything serious is ruled out, it is a question of tackling the headache triggers and, if it is migraine, of using simple painkillers.

THE DIFFERENT TYPES OF HEADACHE

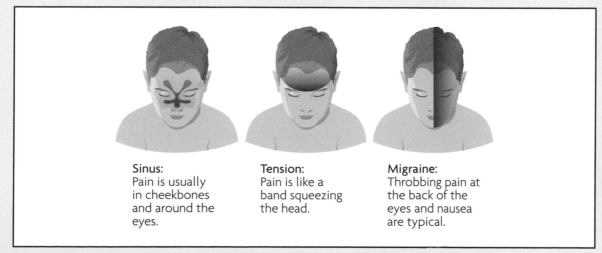

Sinus:
Pain is usually in cheekbones and around the eyes.

Tension:
Pain is like a band squeezing the head.

Migraine:
Throbbing pain at the back of the eyes and nausea are typical.

Always have a follow-up check with the doctor four to six weeks after the first visit.

Tension Headache

- **Find the cause of stress**, if you can, and do something about it. If she is missing school, talk to the teacher to see where the problem lies. Is she being bullied, is she spending long hours on homework or doing too much outside school?

- **Encourage her not to miss school.** Talk to her about her worries and look at solutions together.

- **Reassure her** that the headaches are not serious. Explain how tension headaches work.

- **Don't make painkillers a habit.** If she is regularly taking them already, start winding them down. Try substitute lozenges and she may not even notice the difference.

- **Relaxation exercises**, yoga, massage, outdoor exercise or even hypnosis are much more helpful. Or simply a change of scene.

- **Herbal teas** can be relaxing and are better than caffeine drinks.

- **Watching television** and computer screens and too much texting can make her headache worse.

Migraine

- The best treatment is to abort a migraine attack by **acting as early as you can**. Rest and painkillers are often enough.

- **Act at the very first sign** of a headache. Let her rest in a quiet, darkened room and give her simple painkillers such as paracetamol or ibuprofen.

- **Reduce the lifestyle triggers** where you can. How much time is spent on homework, watching television? What time is she going to bed? (Children with migraine tend to have disturbed sleep so she will need a good bedtime routine.)

- **Anticipate a stressful time**, such as starting school. Look out for early migraine signs. Give her all the reassurance she needs.

- **Cut out any food triggers.** About a third of children with migraine report food triggers, but she may have none. If there is a suspect, try stopping it. The list includes chocolate, citrus fruits, nuts, cheeses, processed meats, caffeine (in soft drinks too), yoghurt, fried foods and monosodium glutamate.

+ She needs to **drink lots of fluids**.

+ **If it is a bad attack** (and if she is over 12 years old) you can sometimes give her nasal sumatriptan.

+ **If she often misses school** because of migraine, your doctor may consider preventive medication. Beta blockers (propranolol) have been studied in children and may be effective, but she should not use them if she has asthma. Anti-epileptic drugs such as gabapentin and topiramate are having encouraging results and may help.

+ **Herbs** (feverfew, ginkgo and valerian root) and vitamins (riboflavin) have been used as alternative or natural remedies for migraine. Feverfew may help migraine, but children should not be given adult doses, and never give it to a child under two years. Capsicum (cayenne pepper) is having some success, but the side effects are considerable and I don't recommend it for children.

+ **Acupuncture** is now a recognised treatment and some people have tried hypnosis, with modest success.

BUT

If headaches get rapidly worse, always call your doctor.

Q&A

Q **She's started getting regular headaches and they've examined her. Now they tell me that everything is normal, but I won't be happy unless they do a brain scan. Why not be absolutely sure?**

A It's hard to be reassured when fears loom large. But if she has had a full neurological examination and nothing has shown up, doctors will not rush to scan or take X-rays. A CT scan will beam as much radiation as 80 chest X-rays and will also be quite frightening for her. Scans can also give a false sense of security. Will there be the same urgency to scan again if the headaches start to change? If there is cause for concern, it will show up in the examination and headache pattern.

Up to 30 per cent of CT and MRI scans happen purely to reassure parents, not because they are needed. A scan is usually advised if a child was previously healthy, now has a headache and has any of these symptoms:

+ A personality change.

+ A neurological and visual examination that is not normal.

- Frequent vomiting.
- A persistent headache which happens when she wakes up, or one that wakes her from sleep.
- Persistent vomiting when she wakes from sleep.
- An EEG (brainwave test) showing focal seizures or focal changes.

Baby Headache

Babies rarely get headaches, though it is very hard to be certain. They do get brain tumours and meningitis. If the fontanelle (the diamond-shaped soft spot at the front of baby's head) bulges, it can be a sign that her brain is under pressure – call the doctor.

Red Alert

HEADACHES I REALLY WORRY ABOUT:

- Your child has a new headache and other symptoms of meningitis (see page 93).
- A headache that happens mostly in the early morning.
- Where she often relieves the headache by vomiting.
- She is also unsteady on her feet.
- Where there is a 'crescendo' headache – more severe and more frequent with each passing week.

Recurring headaches that start to worsen will always concern me. I am less concerned – though the parent may not be – when the headaches have not changed over the past 12 months. These are not likely to be serious.

CT or MRI scans, skull and sinus X-rays are rarely necessary. A neurological examination and the headache history will show abnormalities.

Is It a Regular Stomach Pain?

Just like recurring headaches, a stomach pain that keeps coming back can relate to anxiety (children rarely express their worries in words). Doctors call it recurrent abdominal pain or abdominal migraine and it affects 10 per cent of children at one time or another. It is a very genuine pain, caused by spasm in the bowel, which:

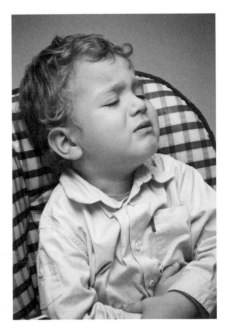

- Is usually around the belly button area.
- Often leads to days off school.
- Does not wake her up at night.
- May be linked to constipation.
- May be quite frequent and severe.

You may feel that she needs some tests to rule out anything serious. But try to avoid the investigation rollercoaster where more and more tests are done 'just in case'. Unless she has **Red Alert** symptoms (see page 219), she really will not need any tests. They may even be counter-productive. Children do not plan it, but all that attention can sometimes reinforce a behaviour pattern that started quite innocently.

She needs a very thorough examination by a good doctor and a lot of reassurance. Not a lot of worrying tests. Above all, she needs to know that she is not 'making up' the pain.

An occasional bad stomach pain can also be caused by constipation, so satisfy yourself that her bowels are in order first. The further the pain is away from the belly button, the more likely there is a physical cause.

Far and away the commonest cause of a regular tummy pain will be abdominal migraine. More rarely, it could be:

- **Inflammatory bowel disease** – she will also have lost a lot of weight, have diarrhoea and very low energy.
- **Coeliac disease** – she will very likely have chronic diarrhoea, a swollen stomach and won't gain any weight.
- **Kidney stones and PUJ obstruction** (narrowing of the tube coming from the kidney to the bladder) – there will be severe pain in the side.
- **Peptic ulceration** – there will usually be a burning pain just below the middle of her ribcage. The pain will be relieved if she takes food or milk.

Home Treatment: Stomach Pains

Always check out a recurring or severe stomach pain with your doctor. If it is recurrent abdominal pain:

- **Look out for stressors.** What has caused the anxiety? A recent event in her life such as a death or moving home? Has she too much schoolwork or outside activities? If there is an obvious reason, try to deal with it openly.
- **Check specifically for bullying** at school.
- **Don't ask about pains** if she has not brought it up. If it hurts, she will tell you.
- **Teach her to deal with pain.** This may include relaxation techniques or holding a warm hot water bottle.
- **Warm herbal teas** such as peppermint, ginger or fennel tea may soothe her stomach and help to relax her.
- **Give her a little paracetamol.** if nothing else works.
- **Encourage her to go to school** if at all possible.
- **Reduce any overload** of homework or extra-curricular activity.
- **Share the good news.** If she has recurrent abdominal pain, make sure that she knows it is good news and a relief for all of you.

Q&A

Q **Her stomach pains can be quite bad and they keep coming back. Could it be a rumbling appendix?**

A I am often asked this but I don't believe in the 'rumbling appendix'. Appendicitis does not recur – it just flares up. If she had acute appendicitis, she would have other symptoms too. She would be miserable, feverish and feel sick and the pain would last for more than four hours. Her stomach would also hurt when you press it gently below the belly button.

Red Alert

TALK TO YOUR DOCTOR ABOUT HER STOMACH PAINS IF:

- She has also lost weight.
- She has regular fevers.
- There is regular diarrhoea.
- She has blood in her stools.
- The pain wakes her at night.
- Pain is not only in the belly button area.

CALL YOUR DOCTOR AT ONCE IF:

She has a new pain that lasts several hours, a temperature and feels (or gets) sick. If the pain is below her belly button to the right, it may be appendicitis. Any pressure on the area will be very sore.

Chapter 19

Sleep Problems

'He's just three and has started waking during the night, maybe three or four times. He keeps appearing at our bedroom door and sometimes I'm so tired that I just take him into our bed. I don't know what's waking him but it can take up to twenty minutes to get him back to sleep. We're all exhausted and now I'm wondering would a sedative help.'

Bed Rage

Sooner or later, your child under four years will develop a sleep problem. Just when you thought you had got through the sleepless stage.

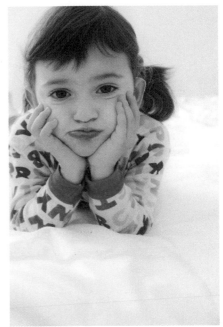

It is not really a problem, except for you, when he is a baby. But by six months, things should start to settle down and it's very tough when they don't.

- ⚕ In eight out of ten cases, the problem is a child who cannot get to sleep without help.
- ⚕ Settling back to sleep can be taught from the earliest age.
- ⚕ In some cases, there may be a physical cause.

It is known in the medical world as 'behavioural insomnia of childhood'. Happily, most sleep problems are short-lived – if they are tackled – and most parents have a great capacity to forgive and forget.

Is It a Sleep Problem?

Ideally, he will follow the natural sleep pattern for his age:

BABIES Newborns can sleep up to 18 hours a day. By six months, it is down to about 14 hours including daytime naps. Newborns naturally wake every four hours or so to feed, but surface briefly every hour. By three months, some babies will naturally start to sleep through the night but it often takes longer.

TODDLERS The sleep–wake cycle gets organised: morning awake, afternoon nap, afternoon awake, night-time sleep. This pattern needs your child to settle to sleep as early as 7 p.m. and to sleep up to 12 hours a day. Naps usually disappear by the time they are three.

SCHOOLCHILDREN Your child sleeps about 10 hours a night and wakes, hopefully, full of energy. Like the rest of us, some children are naturally 'morning' or 'evening' people.

HOW MUCH SLEEP DO CHILDREN NEED?

3–6 years old	10–12 hours per day
7–12 years old	10–11 hours per day
12–18 years old	8–9 hours per day

In reality, the amount of sleep needed varies hugely. I see toddlers who sleep 12 straight hours, with one or two daytime naps – and others who have eight hours of interrupted sleep, with very short naps. None of them has a sleep problem. It is only a problem when they are too tired to go about their daily business and when you find yourself seriously sleep deprived.

If your child is over six months:

- Cries when put to bed.
- Downright refuses to go to bed.
- Wakes during the night.
- Insists on lengthy sleep rituals.
- Wakes for the day at 6 a.m.

And everyone is exhausted, you may have a sleep problem.

Or Something Else?

Sometimes there can be a physical cause for sleeplessness – asthma, sleep apnoea or (very rarely) narcolepsy.

SLEEP APNOEA He is drowsy during the day, breathes through his mouth and his schoolwork is suffering. He wakes often at night and every so often he breathes heavily, then stops breathing for 15 scary seconds or so. He may also sleep in an unusual position and sweat a lot. Snoring is the biggest clue.

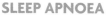

SLEEP APNOEA

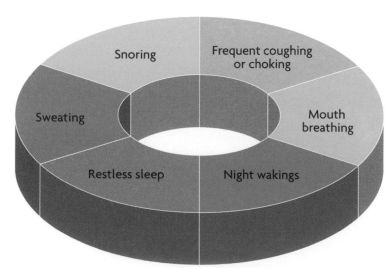

It may be obstructive sleep apnoea, a blocking of the airways. Swollen tonsils or adenoids may be the cause or he may be overweight, have Down syndrome or Pierre Robin syndrome. Doctors will test him (with X-rays and possibly sleep studies) and if adenoids or tonsils are the problem they usually take them out. Sleep apnoea will not kill him but if it's not treated he could have health problems. It often goes unnoticed (a study in 2000 showed that most children were not diagnosed for over three years!), because it usually happens during the early hours when parents are out for the count.

NARCOLEPSY This is serious sleeping; he just cannot seem to get enough of it. Even after 10 hours' sleep at night, he will catnap at the slightest excuse. Stranger still, strong emotions such as laughter or anger will weaken his muscles and make him fall. Narcolepsy often affects obese children but is luckily rare enough. The problem is leaping into REM sleep immediately his eyes close (a sleep EEG will show it), which then spoils his later REM sleep. So he spends his time trying to catch up. It needs specialist testing and is not easy to treat, though stimulants will help.

The Inside Track

Everyone sleeps in cycles: light sleep, deep sleep, REM dreaming sleep. Then a brief waking that we may not even remember, and the cycle starts again. Each adult cycle lasts from 90 to 110 minutes on average and the first REM sleep usually happens about 70 to 90 minutes after we fall asleep. A baby's sleep cycle is much shorter, but by six months it is closer to an adult's and he briefly wakes every 90 minutes or so.

The hypothalamus in the brain is the timekeeper – it reacts to light signals and regulates the timing and length of sleep. Just before falling asleep, levels of melatonin, the sleep-inducing hormone, rise. With adolescents, the timing of release of melatonin moves to a later time at night – which is why teenagers find it hard to sleep before 10.30 p.m.

'Resting' at night is a bit of a misnomer. Your child's brain is just as busy asleep and most of all during REM sleep, when he files experiences into his memory – a very essential process. Adults spend nearly a quarter of the night in REM sleep, while babies need twice as much. But falling asleep is not simple. A sleepy space has to be created and the biggest influences will be his lack of sleep, the circadian rhythm (his body clock) and his bedtime surroundings. We also know that when energy levels drop, the brain releases a chemical (adenosine) as a signal to the body to rest.

Night Waking

Waking up at night is not the problem. Small children naturally surface a few times, open their eyes and move around. Most will fall back to sleep by themselves. The problem is when they cannot settle back to sleep **alone**. It really all hinges on the scene as your child falls asleep. What is happening in your house?

* He always falls asleep downstairs, then you put him to bed.
* He crashes out on the couch watching a DVD.
* You stay with him (maybe even cuddle him) until he falls asleep.
* He always falls asleep on your breast, a bottle or a soother.
* He sleeps in your room and is disturbed when you go to bed.
* He falls asleep with the bedroom light on.
* Bedtime is a rushed, frazzled affair.
* He spends the day in a crèche and has not seen you since breakfast.
* You are over-anxious and pop in regularly to check him, disturbing his sleep.
* He has experienced some trauma (a hospital stay, moving house, new playschool) and is clingy.
* He realises that night time with Mum and Dad is fun.

Sleep studies show time and again that children who fall asleep by themselves are more likely to sleep through the night. It is nice to let him doze off on your shoulder, but ideally his last waking image will be the bed he wakes up in – not you. And night waking should be very boring. If it has any appeal, he would be mad to drop it.

NIGHTMARES AND TERRORS Children start dreaming from an early age and many have nightmares, but fewer have night terrors. Nightmares can be remembered, but night terrors are usually unexplained.

Nightmares happen in the last third of the night, during REM sleep. They usually start at between three and six years of age and your child will wake upset but will be easily comforted. He may be scared to go to sleep for a few nights, however. Nightmares are only an issue if they happen often – maybe once a week – and have the same theme. After a road accident, a child can have recurring nightmares for up to three years and may sometimes need to work with a psychologist.

Night terrors are different. They usually happen about 90 minutes after falling asleep (moving from non-REM to REM sleep) and they will not be remembered. Typically, the child sits up suddenly and screams. He will be very frightened, with dilated pupils and a wide-eyed stare. He may be sweating and have a fast pulse and he may shout gibberish. He will push you away and will only accept your cuddles when fully awake. Eventually – and it could be anything from a few seconds to half an hour – he will fall asleep again. About 5 per cent of children have them, mostly between the ages of three and eleven. While they are very frightening for the parent, they don't seem to bother the child too much.

If he has regular night terrors, you can keep a diary and find when they are most likely (they tend to happen at the same time). Fifteen minutes before a terror is expected, gently wake him. Continue this for a week. It is also possible to block deep slow-wave sleep by using benzodiazepines (sedatives) for a short period, until the terrors stop. This would only be a last resort, however.

HEAD-BANGING, ROLLING AND GRINDING Then there are the acrobats. They are the ones who simply cannot keep still, either just before they sleep or when they drift into light sleep. Rocking and head-banging often start after six months of age. He will roll his head rhythmically from side to side or maybe bang it against the sides of the cot. He may even do it during the night when he wakes, unknown to you. Has he emotional problems? No, nor will he get brain-damaged by it. A lot of children are head-bangers but it would take a far greater force than a small child to cause brain damage. Nobody quite knows why it happens, but most grow out of it by the time they are five. In the meantime, pad the cot sides and ignore it. You can generally ignore teeth grinding too if it starts (it is a habit), but if your child is a serial grinder you can try a plastic mouth guard at night.

SLEEPWALKING He sits up in bed, then – with his eyes wide open – walks purposefully but shakily out of the room. He may babble nonsense as he wanders around. Children have been known to wake up in the street. Like night terrors, sleepwalking is most likely to happen shortly after your child falls asleep, when he moves from non-REM to REM sleep. Over 15 per cent of children sleepwalk and it can start as early as age five, but he will do most of it between ten and twelve years old. It often runs in a family, but don't blame yourself. It is nobody's fault, he is not emotionally disturbed and he will get over it. In the meantime, lock the front door and safety proof his room and the stairs. It is generally better not to wake him.

BEDWETTING This may be disturbing his sleep, but you can help him. (See page 238 for advice on bedwetting.)

Sleep Training

Can you – and should you – train your baby to sleep? The great debate on baby sleep routines continues: does baby or parent call the shots? Do you adopt a 'no tears' approach and respond (with comfort or food) when your baby cries or do you allow him to 'cry down' or cry it out until he eventually settles himself? My advice is to choose the approach that feels right for you. I'm not a great believer in rigid routines for babies, but if you badly need him to sleep through the night they might work for you.

However, it is a different matter when your child is six months old. By now, he should be sleeping through the night and will self-soothe himself to sleep if given the chance. If not, good bedtime routines will make a difference and together with the Controlled Crying Technique you should get a night's sleep.

CONTROLLED CRYING TECHNIQUE Sometimes everything seems to be in place (the routine, the bedroom, etc.) yet he still has a crying fit at intervals during the night. Usually nothing is wrong, except that he has realised that 'When I cry, someone comes'. The controlled crying technique reassures him, but on a sliding scale to the point where crying does not really pay.

- He wakes at 3 a.m. and after gentle crying starts a loud protest.
- Leave him to cry for one to five minutes (depending how much you can take!).
- Go into his room, then lift, cuddle and comfort him.
- When he has calmed to barely sobbing, put him down and walk out.
- He may start crying again immediately. Leave him to cry for two minutes longer than the last time. Then go in and settle him in the same way.
- Once he settles, leave.
- Each time he cries, increase the waiting period by two minutes before you go to him.
- Next day, repeat the process. But this time wait ten minutes the first time he cries, then increase waiting by five minutes.
- You must be firm and both parents must agree to the method.
- Only start if you are ready for a few busy nights. If you follow it to the letter, he should stop crying fits within a week or two. But if anyone diverges from the plan, you will be back to where you started.

Researchers have carried out the first randomised, controlled trial in Australia on six- to twelve-month-old babies with sleep problems, using a strategy of controlled crying, sleep routines and sleeping alone. Within two months, babies (and parents) were sleeping soundly.

Controlled crying works, but I don't believe in it for small babies.

Home Treatment: Sleep Problems

With toddler sleep problems, always look at the evening lifestyle. The best bedtime is a gradual deceleration where he comes off the rollercoaster and is gently nudged into sleep. If your household is buzzing, he will not leave gracefully. And he wants a bedtime routine. It tells him it's time to wind down and it's very reassuring. Everyone has to stick to it, though, or it won't work. But most of all he needs to learn how to fall asleep alone.

If your child is difficult to settle to sleep:

- **Start a sleep diary.** Quite quickly, there is an accurate picture of sleep patterns and bedtime habits.
- **Schedule time** with him before bedtime, if you can.
- **Have a fixed bedtime routine** and commit everyone to it; include grandparents and babysitters. Keep to the same bedtimes. When he is over-tired, everything becomes a fight.
- **You decide** what time he goes to bed, not him – even if he is not sleepy.
- **A sleepy house** makes sleep more attractive. Start to wind him down 20 minutes before you call bedtime. Turn the TV and computers off (until he is gone!), tidy away his toys, lower the lights a little and stop the adrenalin flow. The household should have a haze of calm serenity. Then the ritual starts: bath, toilet, teeth, pyjamas, bedside chat or story, goodnight hug.

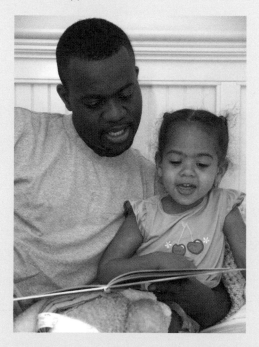

- **Settle him in his own bed.** Put him to bed when he is drowsy, but not asleep. He needs to associate bed with going to sleep.

- **Don't stay with him** until he falls asleep. Leave decisively, when the story is finished. If he is clingy, potter around the bedroom tidying up, but don't talk. Your presence alone will be reassuring.

- **If he appears at the bedroom door**, take his hand and walk him back to bed. And do it again and again (night after night!) if necessary. Firmly and quietly. Conflict won't work – it's attention, isn't it? Set limits over calls for drinks. A sip of water going to sleep should be enough.

- **Keep the bedroom light off**, but use a nightlight if he's anxious. Get him used to noise near the bedroom from the start. Radio playing, doors opening and closing, voices on the landing. You don't want a child who startles if a pin drops.

- **Watch his naps** and avoid evening naps (if you can).

- **Avoid fizzy drinks** (some contain caffeine) in the evening. A bedtime glass of milk is fine, mainly as a sleep signal.

- **A comfort blanket** or scruffy toy may become part of his sleep ritual from the age of 18 months. It can help him to separate from you and the only drawback is the day you lose it. I advise getting two.

- **A sedative may be prescribed** in extreme cases of sleeplessness (usually a tiny dose of antihistamine). I am reluctant to use them but they may help – so long as you also tackle sleep routines. They should be tailed off within weeks.

- **Melatonin** is popular as a natural sleeping aid but it is a hormone and I don't advise it for developing children.

Remember: he probably does want to go to sleep, but if there is a better offer he will take it.

If he wakes during the night and won't settle:

- **Look at the sleep setting.** It's often because something in his environment is different. Did he go to sleep in a different setting or has his sleep trigger (perhaps a bottle) disappeared?

- **Settle him to sleep in his own bed.**

- **Don't take him into your bed** when he appears (try not to!). Walk him back to his own bed.

- **Don't reward night waking.** Make any contact brief and very boring.

- **Minimal talk and eye contact.** If he needs reassuring, your presence will be enough.

- **Avoid sleep triggers** such as a bottle, a soother or a breast.

- **Avoid disturbing him during the night.** Don't change his nappy unnecessarily, and reduce night-time feeds after six months of age.

- **Try controlled crying techniques**, if he's over six months and night wakings are regular.

- ⊞ **If a trauma or major event is the cause**, you may have to take him into your bedroom for a week or two until he's settled.

- ⊞ **Alternate nights** on sleep patrol if there are two of you. It will help you to stick it out.

- ⊞ **If he's an early riser** (wide awake at 6.45 a.m.), you can put him in a low divan bed instead of a cot. He can then get out of bed safely and play with some toys on the ground. But not enough toys to make it exciting. Safety-proof his room and the stairs first.

If you rocked him to sleep at 7 p.m., he will probably want a rocking at 3 a.m. The best scenario is one where you don't figure.

Settling your child in bed when he is drowsy, but not asleep, will help him associate bed with going to sleep

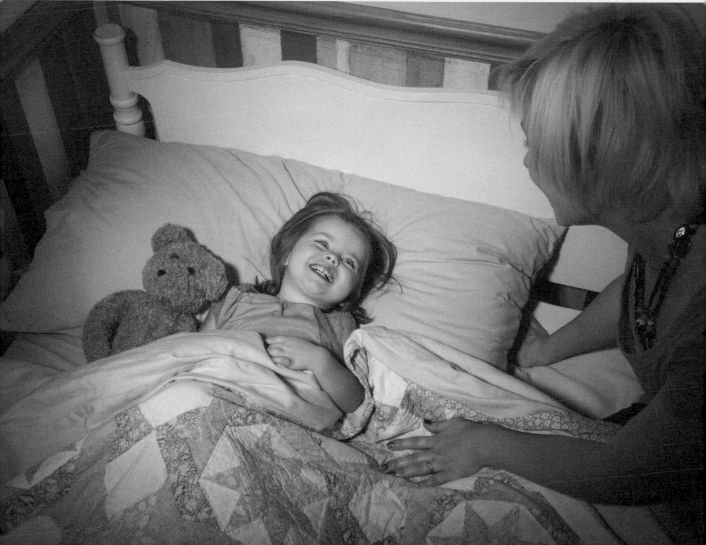

Child's Sleep Diary

		MON	TUES	WED	THURS	FRI	SAT	SUN
Day	**Morning:**							
	time child woke up							
	All naps:							
	time child fell asleep							
	what did you do?							
	child slept how long?							
Evening	**Bedtime:**							
	time child fell asleep							
	took how long?							
	what did you do?							
Night	**1st Night Waking:**							
	time child woke up							
	awake how long?							
	what did you do?							
	2nd Night Waking:							
	time child woke up							
	awake how long?							
	what did you do?							
	Other Night Wakings:							
	how many?							
	what did you do?							

Q&A

Q **Once I get him upstairs to the bathroom, he seems to accept and relax into our bedtime routine. The problem is getting him up the stairs.**

A There has to be something attractive about going to bed. What is your bedtime package and has it a chance against the action downstairs? The challenge is to make bedtime a precious time with you – a time to relax, chat with you about his day, read a story together, have a cuddle. And at the same time, reduce the attractions downstairs where you can.

Q **When he turns up in our room, it's easier to let him into our bed and, to be honest, I like it. It seems perfectly natural, so what's wrong?**

A Cuddling together is the most natural thing in the world and if you do not mind night wakings, go for it. But he will take longer to settle into a sleep pattern. By all means give him a cuddle, but settle him back in his own bed. If he is an early riser and appears at 6.30 a.m. or close to wake-up time, you will not do too much damage bringing him into the bed, so long as your bed is big enough.

Q **Someone told me that if I feed the baby cereal before bedtime, he will sleep through the night. Should I?**

A Many grandmothers will insist that this works, but the evidence from studies is actually conflicting. Introducing solids (i.e. cereals) early is not certain to work and it may cause other problems for a small baby's digestive system. I can't really recommend it.

Q **He's ten and seems a little young to snore, but it's become quite noticeable. What's causing it?**

A He snores because tissues within his pharynx are vibrating or because his nasal airways are blocked. Snoring appears to run in families and he is more likely to snore if you snore too. There also seems to be an allergy link. Studies recently found that children who tested positive for allergies are twice as likely to snore three times a week. Of course, if the child is overweight, he is also more likely to be a snorer.

Snoring is not so unusual and about 20 per cent of children will snore occasionally.

Losing weight (if it is a problem) or sleeping on his side will ease the snores. But snoring is the most common symptom of a medical problem – sleep apnoea – and if it is a regular problem he really needs to be checked out by a doctor or sleep specialist.

Q He had a nasty attack from a dog several months ago and he still wakes up sometimes in a cold sweat. He seems to be having nightmares. What should I do?

A Nightmares can follow any traumatic event and they may last quite a while. Make sure they are not night terrors, though; with a nightmare, he should be able to remember what it was about. Unfortunately, there is no magic cure except a lot of reassurance from you. If they still recur a year later, you may consider talking to a psychologist.

Baby Sleep

🐻 Up to six months, your baby does not have sleep problems. His sleep patterns are erratic because he is feeding and his circadian rhythm is not fully established. If he is breastfed, he is more likely to wake at night.

🐻 I'm not a great believer in strict sleep routines for small babies, but parents can favour either the 'no tears' or 'cry it out' approach to sleep, depending on their needs.

🐻 I do believe in helping baby to learn how to settle himself to sleep, from the start. You can start a bedtime routine from six months:

  ❊ Settle him to sleep in his own cot, when he is drowsy but not asleep. (Sleeping with your very young baby is not a good idea.)

  ❊ Hard as it is, try not to let him fall asleep on the bottle, breast or soother.

  ❊ Always separate day and night for him. Use different cots and different rooms.

  ❊ Make night feeds low-key.

Red Alert

Talk to your doctor if your child has symptoms of sleep apnoea or narcolepsy. He may be referred to a specialist.

Chapter 20

Waterworks & Wetting Problems

'She's six, fully toilet trained and was well settled in her class this year. But now she's started to wet her pants at school. She's very upset about it, yet we can't get her to go to the toilet regularly. We think she has had kidney infections recently and I wonder if they're causing the accidents. Or is something worrying her?'

Wetting & Infections

Wetting is a headache for parents who think they have closed the book on toilet training. Why is she still having accidents, even though she's well out of nappies?

It's a very common problem, but often misunderstood. In most cases, wetting can be solved with a little motivation and a lot of behaviour therapy. But sometimes it can be a sign of infection.

- Bedwetting isn't unusual: 15 per cent of five-year-olds still wet their beds.
- If she is toilet trained, 'holding on' is the most likely cause of daytime accidents.
- 'Holding on' causes urinary tract infections.
- A baby with a urinary tract infection is more likely to have a physical problem.

If you suspect a urinary tract infection, contact your doctor. They are less common in children and need looking into.

Is It a Urinary Tract Infection?

It can be hard to know with small children. Unlike adults, there are no easy clues to an infection. She may be off colour, vomit and have diarrhoea – but there could be other reasons. Her urine won't usually smell much different from normal. And (especially if she is younger) it may not hurt when she goes.

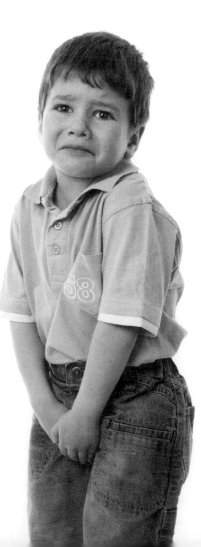

- The best clue is an unexplained temperature.
- If she's under two years old and her temperature is 38°C or more (with no other obvious symptom, such as a sore ear), her urine should be tested.
- An older child may be helpful enough to show some of the classic symptoms: back and stomach pains, a temperature, frequent urinating and blood in her urine.

We need to know why she's infected. Your doctor will send a urine sample for laboratory testing but will also do a dipstick test to get an indirect measure of infection in her urine. If anything shows up, she'll be started on antibiotics as a precaution.

The Inside Track

Her urinary tract is a complex flushing system. It is a cluster of organs (kidney, bladder and the linking tubes, ureters and urethra) that filter out waste from her blood, store it as urine and expel it when she urinates. She learns how to work the system when she reaches full bladder control, normally some time between her third and fourth birthdays. First, sensing when her bladder is full. Then learning to store urine. Finally, wanting to empty (or hold) her bladder at the right times.

Normally, the urine will be sterile. Bacteria do find their way into the bladder – usually *E.coli* bacteria that work their way up from around her anus – but normal peeing flushes most away. Problems start if bacteria have a chance to take hold. This usually happens if urine gets stored for longer than usual, creating a stagnant reservoir. Bacteria start to grow, her organs fight back, becoming inflamed, and she has a urinary tract infection. It is called pyelonephritis when her kidneys are infected; cystitis when it is a bladder infection. A kidney infection is more serious than a bladder infection because there is the risk of damaging the kidneys if it is not treated.

HOW GIRLS' URINE IS PROCESSED

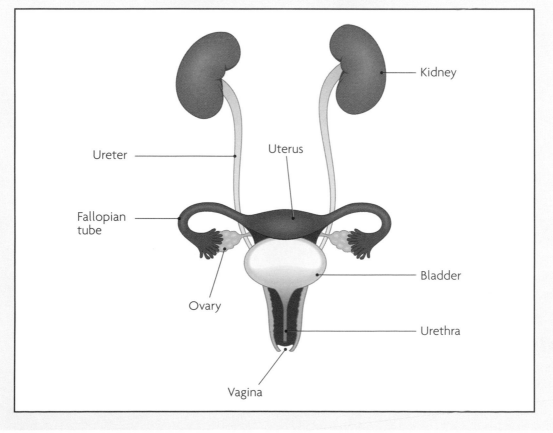

So what causes urine to be stored for longer?

Not drinking enough (ironically). The more she drinks, the more urine she will pass. This flushes the system more often and lowers the chances of bacteria getting a hold.

Physical abnormality. Something traps the urine. It's most likely in a baby under one year old and some 40 per cent of cases will have vesicoureteric reflux (instead of flowing from the bladder down to the exit, the urine 'backs up' and flows up towards the kidneys). Or there may be a blockage somewhere in the system. Some children will turn out to have abnormal kidneys.

Toileting problems. Forty per cent of toilet-trained children who get a urinary tract infection have 'holding on' problems. If she has regular urinary infections, it's almost definitely the cause.

And if you had problems with urinary tract infections, she is more likely to.

Home Treatment: Urinary Infections

Urinary tract infection is one illness that you cannot treat yourself – the risk of damage is too great. She needs a doctor and antibiotics and she will have an ultrasound test of her kidneys. If she's under six months old (or the infection is bad) she will be admitted to hospital for treatment and tests. You can, however, help to prevent future urinary tract infections:

- **Look at her toilet routine.** She needs to urinate at least five times a day and to have enough time to fully empty her bladder.

- **Make sure she doesn't get constipated.** It can encourage her to 'hold on'.

- **Let her drink lots of water** every day, as routine. It will keep her bladder flushing.

- By all means, **get her to wipe herself correctly** after using the toilet. From front to back. It is good hygiene.

- **Cranberry juice** is seen as the natural cure-all. It is thought to deter bacteria, by raising acid levels in the urine, and to stop them sticking to

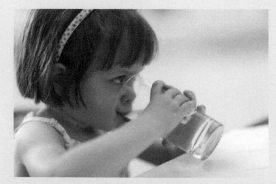

Routinely drinking water every day will help your child's bladder keep flushing

the walls of the urinary tract. It has been successful with urinary tract infections in adults, but there are no clear results yet with children. It is certainly worth trying, but she may not like the taste. Keep doses small, though. Too much can cause diarrhoea.

- **There's no reason to ban swimming.** We know that water (and that includes dirty pool or sea water) does not get into the bladder.
- **Circumcised boys** are less likely to get infected, but before you rush to surgery bear in mind that we would have to circumcise up to 200 boys to prevent one urinary tract infection. It's a significant operation, with risks. It is usually reserved for boys with severe reflux or foreskin problems.

Is It a Wetting Problem?

- It is formally bedwetting (nocturnal enuresis) when she is five and it is all still a problem. She has never been fully dry at night – or she was dry (hallelujah) for six months and has now started bedwetting again.
- Daytime wetting is quite different. She starts to have accidents, just when you though she was toilet trained. There is urgency about the toilet with sudden dashes after a long lull. Often too late.
- Boys are more likely to wet their beds, while girls are almost exclusively the daytime wetters.

The Inside Track

Parents often put bedwetting down to laziness, sleeping too deeply or emotional problems. Very few parents correctly see it as a medical problem and ask their doctor for help. In fact, with the right approach, your bedwetting child will be dry within a few months. Handled wrongly, it can all drag on miserably.

The most important point about bedwetting is that it is involuntary – she's not doing it deliberately. It is a neurodevelopmental problem that does resolve with time, though simple measures will help. Why she does it is a little more complex.

Most children wet their bed because they produce more urine at night than most or have a small bladder capacity. **Some** wet because they sleep too deeply and don't realise they have a full bladder. Of course, she may be genetically prone to it (nearly half of bedwetters will have a parent who did). More recently, researchers have found that a small bladder capacity can also be inherited. In some cases, a stressful event can start her off – an accident, perhaps, or a new baby. But most bedwetting does not have emotional roots.

Normally at night the body increases its levels of an antidiuretic hormone. This makes her kidneys re-absorb more water and so reduces the amount of urine she produces. But some bedwetting children lack this natural circadian rhythm that increases the hormone. And they continue producing daytime amounts of urine. If she wets soon after falling asleep (or if she leaves a large wet area in the bed) this is very likely the problem. She will probably sleep through the whole incident, while a child with a low bladder capacity usually wakes up.

Daytime accidents are usually a problem with toileting routines. Life is too exciting in the playroom or she is not so keen on the school toilet, so she holds on. When she does go, it is a rush and her bladder only gets half emptied. It is quite a serious problem that often goes unnoticed. The big risk is a urinary tract infection.

Home Treatment: Bedwetting

You may decide to do nothing. Most five-year-old bedwetters will eventually solve the problem themselves, but it could be a slow process. If you are more interested in a 'dry campaign' than she is, it is likely to fail.

Try a mix of these treatments for a few months. I advise alarms and medication only if nothing else works.

- ➕ **Throw out nappies** or training pants as she will only cling to them.
- ➕ **Never punish a bedwetting child** unless you want to prolong things. It is not her fault. Better to put her in charge of her 'dry campaign' – and to reward results.
- ➕ **Rule out stress.** A relapse into bedwetting sometimes starts with a stressful event.
- ➕ **Change her drinking routine.** She should take 40 per cent of her liquids in the morning, 40 per cent in the afternoon and only 20 per cent in the evening. Ban drinks with caffeine such as colas; hot chocolate, tea and pure fruit juice can be bladder irritants so avoid them, too. (But don't ban drinks altogether after 6 p.m. as it does not help.)

■ She should go to the toilet **regularly during the day and just before going to bed** — four to seven times daily. If she wakes at night, take her to the toilet.

■ **Try motivating her.** A reward system for dry nights (such as a Star Chart) may help some children over five years old. But keep it going for three to six months.

■ **Light her path.** Make sure she can find the bathroom at night.

■ **Bladder training can also help** — so that she goes only when the bladder is full. Teach her to hold urine when she wants to go, for increasingly longer intervals. You can even test her progress each week with a measuring jug (this method alone will cure 35 per cent of bedwetters).

■ **An alarm clock can work** for some. You wake her after two to three hours of sleep and bring her to the toilet — whether she is wet or dry.

■ **Stay with the new routines** until she is fully dry. It will take months, not weeks.

■ **Always use a protective cover** on your child's mattress, until bedwetting stops.

■ **Alternative therapies** such as hypnosis, psychotherapy and acupuncture can be tried, though studies have shown limited effects on bedwetting.

■ **Use special enuresis alarms.** These have a very high success rate (70 per cent), but work best for children over eight. They work by conditioning. The alarm, which is attached to your child's underpants, goes off when urine is sensed, she wakes and goes to the bathroom to complete the business. After three consecutive weeks of dry nights, it can be stopped. But be prepared to get up several times a night while you're using it and for the first few nights you will probably have to wake her when the alarm sounds. It's best to put her in charge of the alarm. She tests it each night when going to bed, turns it off if it sounds and re-sets it. It will take her longer than desmopressin to reduce bed-wetting — but the effects last much longer.

AN ENURESIS ALARM

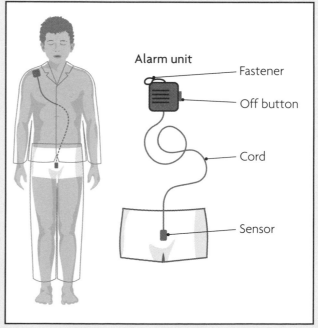

Alarm unit — Fastener
— Off button
Cord
Sensor

■ **Drugs for bedwetting** (such as desmopressin) are only advised if she's over eight and nothing else works. They will reduce the amount of urine she produces at night but children tend to relapse when they stop using them. They can be good for a short-term event, such as a weekend trip or sleepover. If you want a longer-term fix, enuresis alarms are better.

You need to challenge her to work a little to get dry.

Daytime Wetting

Your child really needs to tackle it and not just because of the social effects; 'holding on' can eventually give her urinary infections.

- **Start a toilet routine.** She needs to urinate at least every three hours. Make sure she takes enough time to fully empty her bladder. Try 'double voiding' – get her to try urinating again after she thinks she has finished.
- **Don't let her get constipated.** It will make her hold on all the more.
- **Avoid fizzy drinks.** They can irritate her bladder. Some juices do too – water is always the best drink.
- **Motivate her.** A reward system really helps children who wet themselves by day.

Q&A

Q She has a kidney infection but I'm not happy that they are doing all these hospital tests. Are they really necessary?

A The answer is 'yes', especially if she is under six months. It is very important to find out if she has vesicoureteric reflux – if you don't, she will continue getting urinary tract infections and her kidneys could get damaged. You may also find that there is a kidney abnormality. A small child who gets 'kidney infections' has to be taken very seriously – and babies most of all. If she is over a year old, she may only need an ultrasound, but if anything unusual shows up she will have to do more tests. They can include a MCUG scan of the bladder and a DMSA or MAG3 scan of the kidneys.

Q She's had a few urinary tract infections. Will they cause any long-term damage?

A Not normally. If her infections were caused by a toileting problem and you manage to sort it out the outlook is excellent. She is very unlikely to have damaged her kidneys or bladder. If she has vesicoureteric reflux, though, it is more worrying. The earlier we pick up and treat this reflux, the more chance she has of avoiding any kidney damage.

The biggest worry with urinary tract infection is that the inflammation may scar the kidneys – there is always a 10 per cent chance. This means a greater risk, as an adult, of high blood pressure and even kidney failure. If scans show any kidney scarring, she'll need annual blood pressure checks for the rest of her life.

Q What will happen if they find that she has reflux from her bladder?

A Operations to correct vesicoureteric reflux are less popular these days. This is because giving night-time antibiotics works just as effectively in stopping kidney scars. Reflux usually sorts itself out, unless it is severe and then it may need surgery.

Baby Waterworks

🐻 It's always more worrying when babies have urinary tract infections as they can become very sick. It's immediately suspected if your child under one year has an unexplained temperature.

🐻 Contact your doctor **immediately** if you have any concerns.

Red Alert

TAKE YOUR CHILD TO THE DOCTOR IF:

✚ She is under two, is feeding poorly and has an unexplained temperature.

✚ She is over two and has an unexplained high temperature.

✚ She has regular, unexplained temperatures.

✚ She has a poor flow when she urinates.

✚ She has some of the other classic symptoms of a urinary tract infection (back and stomach pains, regular urinating, and blood in her urine).

The Normal Child

KNOW WHAT TO EXPECT AS YOUR CHILD GROWS

Chapter 21
'Is this Normal, Doctor?' What New Parents Ask

The Common Questions

Knowing what is normal for your child can be difficult — especially if you are a new parent. To help you, I have selected the questions parents ask me most frequently in my clinic.

Q My newborn baby is beautiful and looks normal. But how can I be sure that all is well?

A It's perhaps the most common question of all. Your newborn baby will have been fully examined before he left hospital — a quick assessment after the birth and a formal examination usually on day two. Anything apart from the very unusual should have been picked up before you and your baby went home. The hospital would have told you if they had any worries.

To my mind, the most important part of the hospital examination is the heart (listening for murmurs and feeling the pulses), the hip (hips may be loose or unstable) and the eyes (cataracts, though rare, may be picked up). When I examine a new baby, I always ask about a family history of hip dislocation or heart disease in newborns, as both do run in families. If hip dislocation is in your family, your baby will have a follow-up ultrasound or X-ray. In fact, both hips and heart will be checked again before he is six weeks old.

You might be surprised to know that 3 in 100 newborns do have a congenital problem of some type. But thankfully they are generally mild. The most common problems are undescended testes, cleft lip or palate, heart murmurs, turned-in feet (talipes) or dislocated hips. Minor blemishes such as 'stork marks' are very common and do fade over time.

Q What's the normal weight, head size and length for a newborn baby?

A I'm using metric figures, although some of us still like to know it in pounds and ounces. Because of healthier pregnancies, babies are heavier and longer than 30 years ago — so some grandparents can be surprised.

The average figures at birth are:

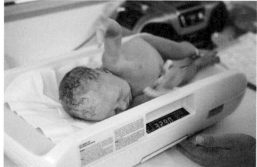

+ Weight 3.5 kg.
+ Length 50 cm.
+ Head size 35 cm.

Keep your own record and fill it out as your baby grows. It really is very helpful to track his progress.

Q My baby has a large head and they are keeping an eye on it. Should I be worried?

A Dad is probably to blame for this, as the vast majority of babies with large heads inherit them from their father. It is really important to have a measurement from birth and then to track his head growth (I advise parents to keep their own record too). If his head was big to begin with (e.g. around 37 or 38 cm at birth) and continues to run on the same percentile line on the chart – then I would not worry. But it does need to be followed up over time. Your doctor will also keep an eye on your baby's development. His head should grow by about 12 cm in his first year of life.

I often see babies with large heads and only get concerned if:

+ The head was normal in size at birth and now is growing very quickly – and the charts confirm this.

+ Your baby's soft spot (anterior fontanelle) is swollen or bulging.

+ Developmental progress is slow.

+ The head is tilted to one side.

+ He has a squint that he did not have before.

Q My doctor has just told me my baby has a slight heart murmur – what does this mean?

A Heart murmurs are very common and mostly innocent. In a young child, the heart rate is double that of an adult and it is very common to get what we call flow murmurs. This is caused by slight turbulence as the blood rushes through the heart. In fact, you will often hear flow murmurs when your child has a fever or if he has anaemia and a low blood count. These murmurs are very soft, do not cause any symptoms and may come and go. They don't need any treatment or precautions.

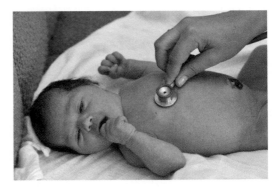

If your baby has a heart murmur, there is little cause for concern. Fewer than 1 per cent of children will have congenital heart disease. Most often it is due to a 'hole' between the two lower chambers (ventricles) and it is called a VSD (ventricular septal defect). If your doctor suspects it, your baby will be referred to a paediatric cardiologist and his heart will be tested by ultrasound or echo. These days, more and more heart problems are, in fact, picked up on antenatal scans. Congenital heart disease does run in families and if you have already had a child with the problem the new baby will be doubly at risk of it.

Q **What should I expect my baby to do by six weeks old?**

A The first six weeks are important and incredible progress takes place in such a short period of time. You should expect your baby to:

+ Have had her first smile!
+ Fix on your eyes and follow them.
+ Respond (by being startled) to loud noises.
+ 'Coo' in response to your voice.
+ Stop crying when she is picked up and spoken to.
+ Have gained 800 grams from birth.
+ Have better head control.

She will still sleep up to 18 hours a day, though patterns will vary. Some babies will sleep for long stretches and others are wakeful. Their tiny temperaments are evident from an early age and a first 'dream baby' is no guarantee of a repeat performance.

Q **My baby's belly button area is sticky – what can I do?**

A This is very common and generally gets better quickly. You can keep the area clean with an alcohol swab (you will find them in the pharmacy) and it should clear up within a week or so. Sometimes there may be a little growth in the belly button area called a granuloma and, if there is, it will remain gooey and sticky despite your best efforts. If so, you will need to see your doctor, who will gently apply a chemical called silver nitrate and tie it off with a simple silk stitch.

Q **My baby's head is very flattened at the back. I've heard about these new helmets – are they worth trying?**

A Baby helmets (for cranial remoulding) have become very popular, particularly in the USA, but I'm not so keen.

Your baby's skull bones do not fuse together until 18 to 24 months and, up to that time, his head shape will reflect the way he lies. We always advise lying babies on their back to prevent cot death so it is no surprise that many babies have temporarily flattened heads. They will right themselves in the end without any treatment. Sometimes your baby may have plagiocephaly (look down at his head and you will notice that his forehead is more prominent on one side than the other). This comes from lying on either the right or left side, but it also resolves with time.

A study in 2014 found that baby helmets were no more effective for flattened heads than leaving everything to nature and time. And parents were not fond of them. The vast majority said that it irritated their baby's skin and most felt that it prevented them cuddling their child.

So avoid helmets – they are an unnecessary expense. If your baby's head is very misshapen from a very early age (soon after birth), it can mean that the sutures of the skull bones have fused early. But this is rare. If you are worried, contact your doctor.

Q **Should I take the baby into our bed? I'm a little worried about cot death.**

A The safest place for your baby in the first six months is in a cot in your bedroom. Save the beautiful new nursery, just for a while. Of course, there's nothing nicer than cuddling up beside him in your bed and you can both enjoy it – when he's awake. But apart from safety, if you want to set up good sleep patterns he really needs to learn to fall asleep in his own bed from an early age. It is dangerous to share the bed with your baby – it is a risk factor for cot death and the risk is higher if either of you smokes, has been drinking alcohol or has taken any drug that makes you drowsy. And it is even more dangerous to sleep with your baby on a sofa or armchair.

Cot death and sudden infant death syndrome is widely researched and studies have found that lying your baby on his back dramatically reduces the risk of cot death (it seems to obstruct the airways less). So does keeping your baby's head uncovered. It's wise to make sure that he can't wriggle down under the blankets – by always tucking him in half way down his cot, with his feet near the end. And don't let him get too hot.

Sleep (apnoea) monitors are a little controversial. They became popular because it was believed that cot death was linked to apnoea, where the baby stops breathing for more than twenty seconds. However, controlled studies have since failed to find a link. But sleep monitors are usually used as a precaution, where there has been any cause for concern.

Breastfeeding appears to reduce the risk of cot death.

Q **My three-month-old baby is ravenous – can I start her on solids?**

A I don't usually advise starting solids until your baby is four months old. If she does seem to be hungry (excessive crying can have other causes, including colic), you could consider changing first to a casein-based formula milk. It will fill your baby better. It's best to hold off solids, so long as she is gaining weight normally. In fact, if you are exclusively breastfeeding you can even delay the introduction of solids until six months old if you want (see page 81).

Q My baby has had a sticky eye for the past two months. What should I do?

A Sticky eyes are very common in babies and are not serious. It's because your baby has tearing mechanisms that are still immature. You will notice a discharge every morning and his eyelids may be hard to separate. The best treatment for a sticky eye is to clean it with cooled, boiled water (with a pinch of salt added) and sweeps of cotton wool from the inside (near the nose) out. Repeat this four times a day for at least five days and eventually it will get better. It's very unusual to find sticky eye persisting and, if it does, you may need to talk to an eye specialist.

Sticky eyes don't need antibiotic drops or ointment. Just daily cleansing. But make sure you see your doctor if:

+ There is a thick and creamy discharge from his eye – and it's there from birth.
+ The eye discharge is bloodstained.
+ The eyelid is very swollen.

Q My toddler has recently started walking and her toes are turned in. Is this normal?

A Toddlers are aptly named because they walk in their own unique way. 'Intoeing' (toes turned in like a pigeon) is very common and is not serious. Her forefoot may be turned in and this is known as metatarsus varus – it's common and will resolve completely without treatment. At worst by the time she is eight years old, but often much sooner. She won't need special correcting shoes because they will make no difference.

Another common toddler sight is the cowboy walk. 'Bowing of the tibia' happens when the bones of the lower leg are slightly bent or bowed. Again, it's not serious and needs no treatment. The cowboy will eventually ride into the sunset.

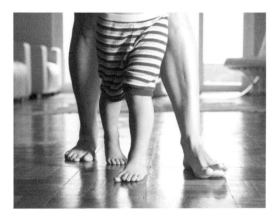

Sometimes, the thigh bone may be twisted forwards and this causes the whole lower limb to twist inwards. But it will correct by the time she is eight years old.

If she has 'knock knees', her knees will be close together. They'll make her fall regularly when she's speeding up, but they're not unusual and don't need any treatment. She will grow out of them.

'Flat feet' are also very common and the best treatment is supportive shoes. Some children have crooked toes and the toes may override each other. Again, supportive, comfortable shoes are all that is needed.

Q He seems to be very clumsy and has problems with the simplest task. Could he have dyspraxia?

A This is a very common question and one that I hear weekly in my clinic. The fancy name for it is developmental co-ordination disorder or DCD. It affects about 1 in 20 children and is more commonly seen in boys. Children with dyspraxia may have trouble writing or riding a bicycle and they may struggle with time management, which affects school performance. They tend to be clumsy and to have difficulty catching objects, using cutlery or participating in sports. Their intelligence is perfectly normal, however. But it's important to know that dyspraxia tends to overlap with ADHD and dyslexia.

You should consider dyspraxia if:

+ Milestones such as walking or speech are delayed. (Many children with dyspraxia have a history of delayed speech.)
+ Other family members have dyspraxia.
+ Your child has ADHD, dyslexia or autism.

There are give-away clues too. I usually ask the child to balance on the dominant and non-dominant leg with his eyes closed and the child with dyspraxia will find this very difficult. He will also struggle with fine motor function tasks such as writing a sentence, writing his own name or using a scissors to cut along a line. What is important is to rule out an underlying neurological problem. These are, thankfully, very rarely seen and I have yet to come across one masquerading as dyspraxia. If a diagnosis of dyspraxia is made, you will need to alert your child's school and look for extra educational supports. Specific tasks (such as cycling) can be improved with practice and some children respond to movement perception training and sensory integration. If the dyspraxia is quite severe, however, your child can be helped by physiotherapists and occupational therapists. His self-esteem may be very brittle and he may be socially isolated – if so, I usually advise some psychological support.

Q My child is a thumb sucker and a nail biter – any suggestions?

A Up to one-quarter of young children nail bite or suck their thumbs. Thumb sucking is normal in babies and nothing to worry about. But it's not ideal if it continues beyond three years of age as it can interfere with teeth alignment. Sucking tends to ease off with time but if you are anxious to stop it the best strategy is a substitute – perhaps a comfort blanket or teddy.

Nail biting is almost universal and is a difficult habit to break. Some parents finally resort to using a bitter-tasting nail varnish which may break the habit. (When nail biting is excessive, it can be a sign of tension in a child.)

This also raises the soother debate. About half of parents use soothers (or dummies or pacifiers, depending where you live). They help to calm a baby if feeding is inconvenient and they do satisfy the sucking needs of babies. There is even some evidence that soothers may help to slightly reduce the risk of cot death – because alertness levels may be higher. But you should aim to get rid of the soother once she is one year old as it can affect her teeth alignment and bring business in the way of your orthodontist. The effects on speech are not as clear, but a soother will certainly stop her experimenting with sounds as she should. The best way to stop the soother is to get rid of it. But she will need a substitute, the same as a thumb sucker.

Never dip soothers in sweet liquids as this plays havoc with your baby's teeth.

Q I've noticed that he has lumps in the neck. Is it serious?

A This is very common and causes parents a lot of anxiety, but it is not usually serious. Swollen lymph glands in the neck are most often linked to a cold or sore throat – the glands are busy fighting an infection. If he has had a bout of tonsillitis, the glands at the front of his neck may have swollen, but they will settle down again after two to four weeks. Glandular fever can cause swollen neck glands too, but he will also feel very tired and lethargic, may have a high temperature and there may be swelling in his groin.

If you are at all worried, please see your doctor. I worry about lumps when I see these signs:

+ The lumps are firm, fixed and **very** large (bigger than a table-tennis ball).
+ There are night sweats, fever or weight loss.
+ There are gland lumps somewhere else.
+ He is a very pale, anaemic child.
+ There are signs of bruising.

The vast majority of children with lumps in the neck have simple lymph gland swelling caused by a viral infection. These are of no concern.

Q **She's one and a half years old and is very pale – is it anaemia?**

A Up to 10 per cent of toddlers are anaemic (they have a low blood count). If your child is anaemic, she will be 'Casper' pale, cranky, off form and prone to infections.

In the vast majority of cases it is a lack of iron and is diet-related. Remember that, no matter how well she is growing, if she drinks too much cow's milk she can become anaemic; it tends to leave less room for the right foods. A blood count test will confirm if she has anaemia but you really need to catch it early as a severe lack of iron can affect how her brain develops. If you also notice blood in her stools, tell your doctor. (See page 179.)

Q **My child has leg pains and people tell me that they're probably just growing pains. Are they right?**

A Leg pains are very common in children and usually have very little to do with growing. Typically, he has leg cramps at night (mainly the lower legs) and they can be quite painful. The pains affect both legs equally but will not make him limp. This is usually a sign of a child who is extremely loose-jointed and active – he uses his muscles more than most during the day, they get weary and when he stops to rest they get cramped. It is known as joint hypermobility and the best treatment is simple massage. A warm hot water bottle on the legs and a mild painkiller will help if it really bothers him. Children with it are more prone to cramps and injury and, for some, it is an argument for keeping children under ten away from contact sports.

I would only worry about leg pains if his joints are also swollen or if he seems very unwell.

Q **She has started to limp recently but I don't really know why. Should I be worried?**

A You need to see your doctor. Any child with a limp should be checked out and watched. There may be a reason – a twisted ankle or a sore foot from a knock – but if nothing seems obvious it needs a closer look.

Has she started school yet? If not, and if it started with a sore throat or a cold, it is most likely inflammation of the lining of her hip joint. It will settle with rest and painkillers over a few days.

Most limps are not serious and last a few days. Some need a doctor:

+ If she also has a high fever and is clearly quite sick.
+ If the limp lasts longer than a few days or keeps coming back over weeks (it may be Perthes disease and she will need orthopaedic help).

+ If joints are also swollen and tender for more than six weeks (it may be childhood arthritis).

+ If she is a teenager starting puberty and is a little overweight (she needs orthopaedic help **urgently**).

Q My child has a lot of bruising over his lower legs. Is this normal?

A Bruising, especially when it's on the front shin, is very normal in active, tumbling young children. If your child has big bruises somewhere else, though, you need to check if he has had any recent falls and see if it all fits.

If there is a lot of bruising, or if it happened after a relatively small knock, then consider other possibilities and contact your doctor. I worry about:

+ Fresh bruising with a fever and pinpoint spots that do not fade under pressure. (Could it be meningitis?)

+ Multiple bruises on a pale child.

+ Bruising with a bleeding nose or mouth, yet no obvious incident that caused it.

+ Bruising over the back of the thighs in a child who seems well but who may also have tummy cramps and joint swelling.

+ Bruising in unusual places. Physical abuse does happen, I'm afraid.

Most bruising, however, is not serious. It is the sign of a busy child.

Q She's six and always seems to be coming down with colds. Is anything wrong?

A Probably not. Remember that the average child gets up to eight colds a year – and they cluster in the same winter months. If she has recently started school, she will have more colds than ever. But a cold should last two to three days at worst. If the child is iron deficient she will be more prone to them, so make sure she is eating iron-rich foods. Disorders of the immune system are exceptionally rare (the commonest, IgA deficiency, affects 1 in 400 people). But if her symptoms get worse, or other problems appear, talk to your doctor.

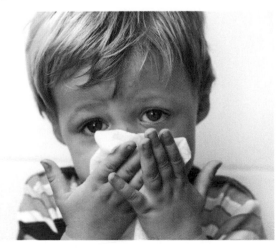

Q My toddler is having terrible temper tantrums – what should I do?

A Unfortunately temper tantrums are a normal part of toddler life, especially between the ages of 18 months and three years. Some toddlers may even breath-hold as part of the tantrum and this is frightening to watch. It is very difficult, but you must remain calm throughout. The best policy is 'time out' – send your screaming toddler for a five-minute time away to cool off. But you must make sure that he does not escape early and that both parents (and even grandparents) all stick to the plan. Consistency is the key and the phase will pass. Biting and hitting fellow toddlers are also possibles, but this is usually a short-lived stage. Do remember that tantrums usually come out of frustration or a need for attention. Try not to reward him with attention but nip frustration in the bud where you can. Especially when there is a pattern to his tantrums.

Q She tends to stutter when she speaks. Should I worry?

A This is really not unusual. In fact, about 1 in 20 children may stutter. They will tend to repeat a sound or may stop talking altogether, with a pause that seems to last for ever. Then they often start to avoid certain words (the words that set off the stammer) and opt out of speaking out in class for fear of embarrassment.

It can become very distressing for them, but most children will outgrow the problem. Many will have mild stuttering when they get excited or angry, usually repeating sounds or words. It is all part of learning to talk and they get clearer as they develop fluency.

If she is under eight years old, I recommend that you don't complete sentences for her or correct her speech. A patient listener is best. When she stutters, reassure her that it's a normal part of learning to talk. She needs an environment that encourages relaxed speaking. In older children, there is a technique called 'syllable timed speech' which is taught as part of an intensive course and is successful. Most children will outgrow a stutter, but if it persists for up to a year she may need help. I will normally refer a child to a speech and language specialist when:

+ 10 per cent or more of her speech has stuttering.
+ She stutters in most situations (not just when she is tired or upset).
+ Speaking embarrasses her or makes her anxious.
+ There are physical symptoms when she speaks, such as blinking eyes.

Q This is my child's fourth bout of tonsillitis this year. Should his tonsils come out?

A Tonsillectomies have largely gone out of fashion. It is not a minor operation so it should be 'earned'. First you need to confirm that it's always tonsillitis. Is there a high temperature, a very sore throat, general misery? Your doctor should find white spots on the tonsils each time. The main reasons for taking out tonsils these days are:

+ An abscess on the tonsils, which is rare but incredibly painful. (You never want to experience it a second time!)

+ Kissing. Very enlarged tonsils that meet in the middle and just touch (are kissing) each other are often associated with large adenoids. It may all make his breathing erratic at night and make him snore loudly. This sleep apnoea is a reason for taking out both the tonsils and adenoids.

+ Regular bouts of acute tonsillitis, confirmed by your doctor.

Your child's tonsils are there for a good purpose – do not push to have them removed unless it is really necessary. And recurring tonsillitis does not make your child chesty.

Q I've been told that my baby has 'tongue tie' and I'm worried that it will cause problems for her.

A Tongue tie (ankyloglossia) is quite common in babies and children. The piece of skin that joins the tongue to the floor of the mouth is short, or taut, so the tongue movement is restricted. It does not seem to interfere with normal development of speech. If your child has tongue tie, but can still stretch her tongue to her lower lip, she will not need an operation to release it.

Chapter 22

The Normal Stages of Development

When Will It Begin?

The rate at which babies learn new skills will vary a good deal – even within the same family. Some will even miss out on a stage, crawling being a classic example. But your child should reach the different developmental stages within a broad timetable.

The rate of development will depend on how quickly his nervous system matures, which is largely genetic. But it will also be influenced by the amount of stimulation he gets, from you or his carers – especially in those early years, when he soaks up information and experiences like a sponge.

Parents tend to worry most about motor development. When will he sit up? When will he walk? In fact, fine movements (grasping and manipulating) and speech are much more likely to influence your child's potential.

This chapter shows you what, generally, normal development is.

Newborn

Your new baby will be very floppy, but his body will react in a certain way. When you hold him with your hands under his stomach, his head will drop down but his arms and legs will be slightly flexed. When you pull him to sit, his head will fall back. Hold him in a sitting position and his back will curve, while his head will fall forward. If you lay him on his stomach, his head will promptly turn sideways. When laid on his back, his arms and legs will flex slightly – quite symmetrically. This is all very normal.

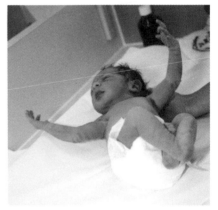

The 'Moro reflex'

He will have primitive reflexes and they are really quite fascinating. The 'Moro reflex' is perhaps the best known. It's a startle reflex – he will react to a seeming fall or sudden noise by immediately splaying his arms and opening his hands. Then his arms come together again like an embrace. From birth, he will react with a startle to loud sounds and his eyes may turn towards a voice.

Other instincts are there from the start. If you hold him with his feet on a firm surface, he will make primitive stepping and walking movements. Rooting and sucking are also instinctive. If you rub his cheek, he will turn his face to find your finger and when you put your finger in his mouth he will suck it. During the first four or five months, he will also have an instinctive grasp. Put your finger in the palm of his hand and he will grab hold of it.

Newborn babies can see and hear. And within a few days of his birth, he will be aware of you, when he is awake. But he will sleep up to 18 hours a day.

BUT

If your newborn baby seems slow to respond, talk to your doctor.

Sitting and Walking

Most children follow through the same stages to sitting and walking – but may get there at different ages.

Lack of opportunity can be an issue. He will be slower to sit and walk if he cannot move around freely. Is he left in his cot or buggy too long and is there enough stimulation to motivate him to move? Ironically, baby walkers slow progress because babies can be left in them for too long.

Over 90 per cent of babies will begin to sit without support between 6 and 11 months. By six months they will stand with support. They will crawl between 6 and 12 months, walk alongside furniture from 8 to 13 months and walk by themselves by the age of 18 months. At this stage, they will climb onto a small chair without help and walk up the stairs holding one hand. A small number may skip the crawling stage and move directly from sitting to beginning to stand and walk.

These babies find bottom shuffling very effective and they can certainly fly along. It is not a problem, though it may delay the time when they start walking (up to two years old).

Your ethnic group can cause some variation. For example, babies of African origin tend to walk at an earlier age (many as early as nine months). And if your baby has high muscle tone or floppiness, he will reach these motor milestones either faster or slower.

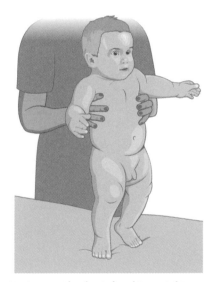

At six months, he takes his weight on his legs when standing

BUT

If your child is not walking by 18 months, talk to your doctor.

Vision

Newborns do not all have the same visual responses. It often depends on how naturally alert they are. But there are some standard reactions. Within a few days of birth, if you hold your child upright he will turn his eyes towards any large light source. And close them if there is a sudden bright light.

During his first month of life, he will stare at objects close to his face. He will show special interest in the human face (his food source) and will follow slow movements of a face, especially his parents'. His first defensive blink will appear from four to six weeks of age.

By six weeks, your child will fix on your face and turn his eyes to follow your face when you move it slowly in a quarter-circle. A squint is not unusual when he is still a few months old, but it is definitely abnormal if he has it at six months. Between two and three months, he should follow a moving light with his eyes.

At six months, he will look at (and fix on) a small 2.5 centimetre block from 30 centimetres away.

By nine months, he will look at (and poke) small objects such as crumbs from the same distance.

By one year, he will point to objects that he wants and when he is out and about he will watch people or animals with intense interest.

Testing his vision when he is under three years old is difficult and needs a trained person. From age three, testing is easier.

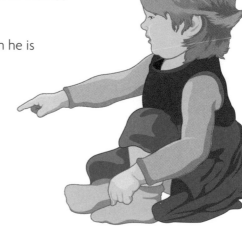

At 12 months, your child can point out desired objects

BUT

If he does not fix his eyes on your face or if his eyes seem to wander by six weeks, talk to your doctor.

Fine Movement

During his first year, he learns how to hold objects. By four months he can hold and drop an object, but cannot pick it up if it falls. Then he works out how to approach an object and grab it with the two palms of his hands – a very crude grabbing hold, usually at six months. He will also be able to move the object from hand to hand. Then he learns how to refine it all until at one year he has perfected the 'pincer grasp' and can pick up a crumb using the tip of the thumb and forefinger. By 15 months, he will build a tower of two toy blocks and by two years he will turn a door handle.

By three years old, most children can hold a pencil between their first two fingers and thumb, using the preferred hand. By four years old, they can cut out a picture with a scissors and start to throw a ball overarm. Hand dominance starts to become obvious around 18 months old and 80 per cent of children will be naturally right-handed.

His self-feeding should also progress. At one, he should drink well from a cup with little help from you, hold a spoon and try to use it to eat. By two, he will lift and drink from a cup without spilling and over the next few months will start to eat well with a spoon and maybe use a fork.

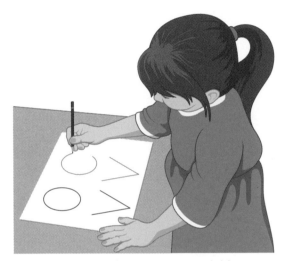

At three years, your child copies a circle and the letter 'v'

BUT

If he is slow to grasp and hold objects, talk to your doctor.

Hearing

He will be startled by loud sounds from the very start and his eyes may turn towards the source. By one month, he will notice a continuous sound. By four months, he will always turn towards a nearby sound and will soothe or smile at the sound of your voice. By six or seven months, if you speak he will turn to you immediately and look at you. By nine months, he will hear very quiet sounds made out of sight, and try very hard to locate them.

Newborns are now screened for deafness in many countries and if a newborn has nerve deafness he is referred for hearing aids or (later) for cochlear implants. The distraction test is no longer routine at nine months.

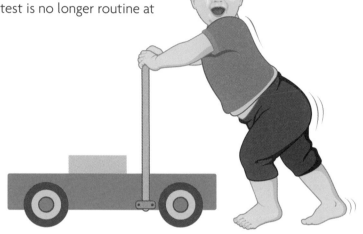

At twelve months, he responds immediately to his own name

BUT

If you are concerned that he can't hear, talk to your doctor; especially if he is not responding to loud noises or seems startled when you appear at his cot. If you have a family history of deafness, say so.

Speech

You will hear his first attempts at language at around six to eight weeks: those 'cooing' sounds we all love to hear. These sounds soon build up until you start to hear vowels and consonants. At about four months, the babbling starts and he makes sounds like laughter. His babbling then gets increasingly complex and (towards the end of the first year) you start to hear strings of syllables such as 'mama' or 'papa'. From six to nine months, he may start to associate one or two words with objects or he may respond to simple phrases like 'bye-bye' or 'clap hands'. He will imitate sounds and actions – and enjoy hearing his own voice!

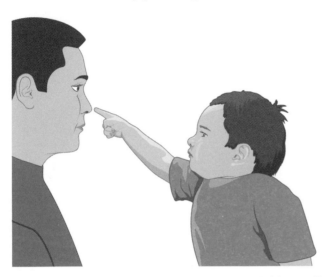

By one year, most children will respond to simple commands

From 10 to 14 months, he really starts to express himself. Now he has primitive words to show his likes and dislikes and his demands. Or 'pre-words' such as 'dis', 'da', 'na'. Some children have one or two basic words by their first birthday. Gradually all the babble, pre-words and gestures build up into a recognisable spoken vocabulary.

But the age at which he first uses a real word is very personal and variable (do not compare him with his big sister). Often baby's first word is 'Dada', much to the dismay of his devoted mother. But 'Dada' is just easier to say than 'Mama' – it's as simple as that.

By one year, most children will recognise names of some everyday objects without the help of clues and respond to simple commands. During their second year, they quickly build up a vocabulary and can respond to two sentence commands. By two, most will have two-word 'sentences' (though 10 per cent will be slower and may not get there until they are three). By three, they can make short sentences and by the age of four, your child should be able to retell a simple story. He should also be generally intelligible to strangers. By age four, he usually has a vocabulary of around 1,000 words, can use the past tense and five-word sentences easily – and may also know some bad language!

BUT

If his speech seems to be badly delayed, talk to your doctor.

Social Behaviour and Play

Within a few days of his birth, he will be aware of you or anyone who cares for him. He will look at you and his expression will change – those first little communications are fascinating to watch. But he will not start smiling at you until he is between six and eight weeks (any earlier grins are simply wind).

At four to six weeks, if you pick him up and speak to him he will stop crying and will turn to look at your face. By three months, he will stare unblinkingly at your face when he feeds. He will also start to enjoy playful tickling and funny sounds you make and by the time he is six months old, he will be delighted when you play with him. At this stage, he won't 'make strange' with anyone but he may start to worry if you are out of sight.

From nine months, however, he knows a stranger and will be very wary of their advances. He will play 'peek-a-boo' and will copy you when you clap your hands. By one year, he will wave goodbye and begin pretend play. He will be quick to look for, and find, a hidden toy. But he will not want you (or those he knows) out of sight or hearing.

By 15 months, he will push a large, wheeled toy with a handle and will carry dolls (by their limbs or hair!). This is when the Danger Age starts: he is exploring his world and you really cannot leave him on his own – exhausting though that may be.

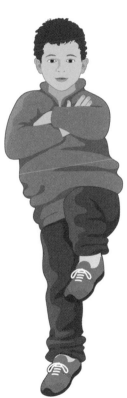

Now his playing becomes more creative. At 18 months, he will happily play by himself but still likes to be near a familiar adult or older sibling. He will listen to stories and look at the pictures. Then by two years, you will notice 'make-believe' play (it's wonderful to watch) and he will play near others but not with them. He will happily play with other children by the time he is three and enjoy 'make-believe' with them. At age four, he will sing simple songs and often have an imaginary friend. And by the time he is five, you will see elaborate make-believe games with his friends.

You may need to get advice if his play is very repetitive or if he is not responding to your attempts to play.

At five years, he stands on one foot and folds his arms

It is a fascinating journey and you will be mesmerised by it all – enjoy it!

Source: Based on recognised guidelines by Mary D. Sheridan, *From Birth to Five Years.*

Chapter 23

The Safe Child & the Top Six Causes of Injury

Reducing Injuries

This book is all about childhood illness. But since the health of children is our concern in writing the book, we cannot ignore accidents. The fact is that more children damage their health through injuries, in the home or outside, than from any illness.

These guidelines aim to keep things in balance. We have drawn on the joint knowledge of paediatricians across Europe, who treat children's injuries daily, to help you keep your child safe.

Reducing the risk of injury is surprisingly straightforward.

No. 1: Road Accidents

The problem: Serious injury in car or cycling accidents.

The solution: Child restraints or child car seats – and bicycle helmets.

Car accidents are the number one cause of death and serious injury for children. If your child has a special car seat or child restraint, you reduce his chances of injury by 90 to 95 per cent (if rear-facing) and by 60 per cent (if forward-facing); **as long as you use it properly**. Car manufacturers may well build in child restraints in the future, to make them as easy to use as seat belts.

THE DIFFERENT STAGES OF CHILD CAR SEATS

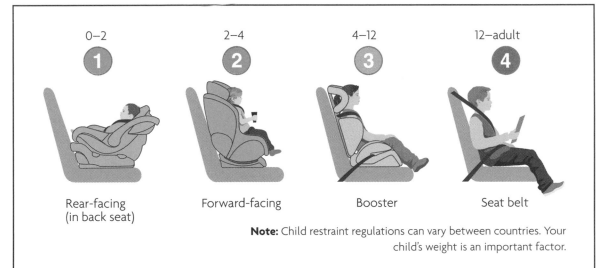

| 0–2 | 2–4 | 4–12 | 12–adult |
| 1 | 2 | 3 | 4 |

Rear-facing (in back seat)   Forward-facing   Booster   Seat belt

Note: Child restraint regulations can vary between countries. Your child's weight is an important factor.

If he cycles, a helmet reduces his risk of head and brain injury in an accident by at least two-thirds, but only if he fits it correctly.

If you can, encourage your local authority to set up traffic calming near your home. It can save children in your area from being knocked down by passing cars. Calming has reduced road injuries in 30 kph zones very dramatically — by 60 per cent.

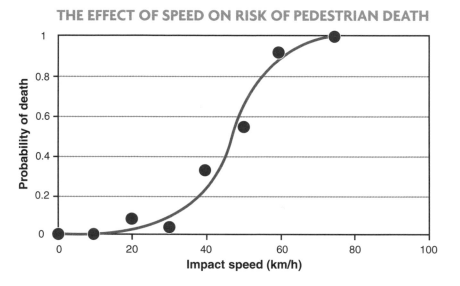

THE EFFECT OF SPEED ON RISK OF PEDESTRIAN DEATH

No. 2: Drowning

The problem: Boating and water accidents.

The solution: Always wear a lifejacket or personal flotation device.

Every year, 85 per cent of drownings from boating accidents could be prevented, if the victim had been wearing a lifejacket. It is the second leading cause of death in Europe. Unfortunately, small boys are most at risk (over 70 per cent of victims are boys) and the most likely age is from one to four years old. What does he wear when he potters around in that old rowing boat?

The problem: Drowning in a swimming pool.

The solution: Isolation fencing for private or holiday pools.

If you are holidaying somewhere with a private swimming pool — or are lucky enough to have one at home — make sure it is fully fenced off with self-latching gates. Fencing a private pool gives 95 per cent more protection against drowning. But no fencing can replace parental supervision! Agree clear and simple safety rules about using any pool. And be careful with garden ponds — even the shallowest pond can be dangerous if a small child falls in.

Teach your children to swim from the earliest age; they can learn from the age of two years. But always keep close watch. Never leave children alone near water.

Red Alert

EMERGENCY AID FOR NEAR-DROWNING:

➕ You must get him breathing, as quickly as possible.

➕ If he stops breathing, give him mouth-to-mouth resuscitation immediately.

➕ Send someone for medical help if you can, but **don't stop** the resuscitation.

➕ Keep it going for as long as you can. Breathing can start again more than one hour after it has stopped.

If your child is breathing, but unconscious, put him in the 'recovery position' (lying on his side). (See page 106.)

Resusitation (CPR)

➕ Hold your child's head tilted back (so you can look into his nostrils) and pinch his nose closed.

➕ Take a deep breath and cover his mouth with yours – making a seal. Breathe into his mouth. Give five of these rescue breaths to start.

➕ Then give 30 'chest compressions': press down with the **heel** of your hand (no fingers!) in the middle of his chest, just above the angle of his ribs. Then release, keeping your hand on his chest. They should be quick presses, more than one per second.

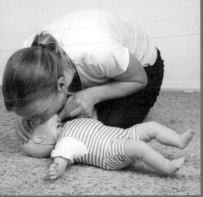

How to carry out mouth-to-mouth on a baby

➕ Now alternate two rescue breaths with 30 compressions, until his breathing starts again.

➕ If he is a baby, cover his mouth and nose with your mouth during rescue breaths. Use two fingers only for compressions. It's **very important** not to tilt your baby's head too far back.

Continuous chest compression (CCR) is the newer, modified form of CPR but it is not suitable for drowning cases or for children under eight years old.

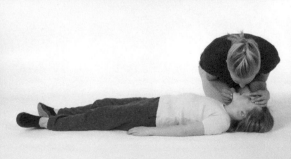

How to carry out mouth-to-mouth on a child

No. 3: Burns and Scalds

Your toddler under two years old is most at risk. Do your children know the basics of fire safety? They will remember most if they learn through demonstration – local fire stations are very good at getting the message across.

The problem: Cigarette lighters and cigarettes.

The solution: Child-resistant cigarette lighters.

If you or someone in your house smokes, use a cigarette lighter that is child resistant. They have been developed and successfully tested and you can even find self-extinguishing cigarettes. In the USA, fire deaths from cigarette lighters dropped by 43 per cent when child-resistant designs were adopted. In 2014, the EU confirmed its ban on novelty lighters and required all lighters to be child resistant – but be careful with holiday buys.

The problem: Scalding water in taps and hot drinks.

The solution: Pre-set temperature for all water heaters – and mind your coffee.

Set your household water heater at less than 54°C. This has proved to be the safest way of reducing hot-water scalds. And when you have a cup of tea or coffee put the milk in as soon as it is poured. Never hold your child on your lap while you are having a coffee and use kettles that have a short flex.

The problem: Household fires.

The solution: Smoke detectors in the home.

Detectors really are a 'must' in any home. The early warning helps to reduce house fires by 71 per cent and they are compulsory under law in new homes and rented properties. Make sure they are installed properly, though, and always test the batteries regularly (don't take the batteries out if your toaster tends to smoke). If you have open fires, have you a childproof fireguard?

The problem: Sleepwear that is inflammable.

The solution: Buy non-inflammable pyjamas and sleepwear.

In the USA, legislation has been very effective; since 1972, when it was introduced, there has been a 75 per cent drop in admissions to hospital burn units for burns from inflammable sleepwear.

The problem: Fireworks.

The solution: Don't!

Firework injuries can be very serious and disfiguring and the only way to reduce them is to ban fireworks completely – starting in your home.

Red Alert

EMERGENCY AID FOR BURNS AND SCALDS:

Bring him immediately to a cold water tap. Run plenty of cold water over the scald or burn (not at full pressure). Do this for at least 10 minutes to reduce the heat in the skin.

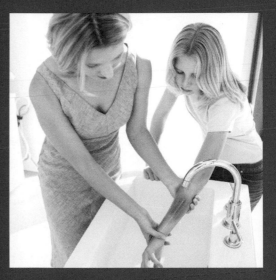

- Remove hot clothes that **are not** stuck to his skin. But **don't** remove any clothing that is stuck.
- Take off socks, gloves or jewellery if feet or hands have been burned. Burned skin can swell up.
- After cooling his skin under the tap, cover the burn. Use a clean cloth (must be non-fluffy) soaked in cold water. This helps to protect the damaged area and will reduce the risk of infection.
- Call an ambulance or take him to hospital yourself.
- Never prick any blisters that develop.
- Don't put butter or any fatty substance on a burn – and no ointments, please! They will have to be cleaned off before the burned area can be treated.

No. 4: Falls

The problem: Falls down stairs or from high windows.

The solution: Stair gates and safety locks on upstairs windows.

Up to 50 per cent of toddler injuries are caused by falls. Falling downstairs can be prevented with stair gates, ideally at both the top and bottom of stairs. Windows are very dangerous: most children who are seriously injured or killed from falls will have found an open window upstairs. Balcony falls are luckily less common because of new building regulations, but be careful on holidays. And be wary of baby-walkers – they are still popular but they have been shown to be dangerous because babies fall downstairs and even steer them into fires. Luckily, playgrounds these days are much safer places and serious falls there are less likely, thanks to absorbent surfaces and safer equipment.

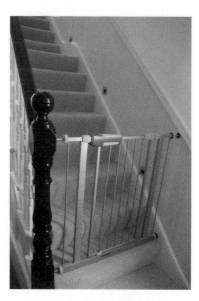

Red Alert

EMERGENCY AID FOR FALLS:

- Check the important things: is he conscious, is he breathing and is there any bleeding?
- If he has stopped breathing, give him mouth-to-mouth resuscitation (see page 267) and get emergency help.
- If he is unconscious or very drowsy, put him in the recovery position (lying on his side).
- If you think he may have a broken limb or an internal injury, **don't move him** unless you absolutely have to.
- If you feel he is seriously injured, dial 999 and call an ambulance.
- If he is drowsy, limp or pale after a fall (or vomits and seems dazed), bring him immediately to your doctor or hospital.

No. 5: Choking

It's nearly always the small, attractive objects that make a child choke: bits of toys, balloons, small pieces of food. But equipment causes choking too.

The problem: Cribs, cots and equipment that can trap.

The solution: Choose baby equipment very carefully.

Safe equipment (and laws that oblige manufacturers to design safely) do more to prevent choking than any vigilant parent. Check his cot or buggy for choking risks and safety compliancy.

The problem: High-risk products such as:

- Latex balloons.
- Pull-cords on windows (e.g. blinds).
- Drawstrings on children's clothes.

The solution: Keep them out of your house.

These are the ones that cause most problems and there are moves to ban them by law.

Red Alert

EMERGENCY AID FOR CHOKING:

- Don't waste time trying to get hold of the object he is choking on, unless it is very easy to reach. It will usually be too far back.
- Hold him upside-down by the legs (if he is a baby or toddler).
- Slap him smartly between the shoulder blades with the heel of your hand. If the object does not fall out, **do it again**. If he is too big to hold upside-down, lay him face downwards across your knees.
- **Don't** use the Heimlich technique on young children. It may promote vomiting and can damage internal organs.

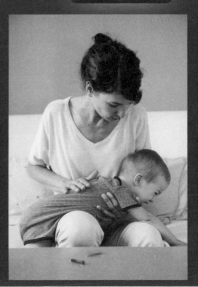

No. 6: Poisoning

Children under two years old will swallow anything to hand – they are the ones who get poisoned. And 90 per cent of the time, poisoning happens at home.

The problem: Common household products such as:

- Cleaning supplies
- Alcohol
- Pesticides
- Medicines
- Cosmetics.

The solution: Store them out of reach and use child-proof locks on cupboards.

Red Alert

EMERGENCY AID FOR POISONING:

- Give him sips of water and **don't** try to make him vomit.
- It may be hard to know for sure if he has swallowed something – but always have him checked out.
- Take a sample of the suspect poison or medication (and its container) to your hospital or doctor. If he vomits, take a sample of that too.

These child safety guidelines have been endorsed by the Child Accident Prevention Committee of the European Academy of Paediatrics, of which the author is a member.

Chapter 24

How to Grow Normal Teeth

Protect Your Child's Smile

Teeth are a health concern but they are often overlooked during a child's early, important years. If you want your child to have a healthy adult smile, please look after her teeth. Unfortunately, she can do a lot of damage before she visits the dentist for the first time.

Remember that:

- Fillings caused by tooth decay are **not** inevitable.
- 'Baby bottle tooth decay' is very real.
- Sugared drinks are the main cause of decay.
- Dental sealants can reduce her chances of decay by up to 80 per cent.

I would always advise bringing a child to the dentist **before** she develops teeth problems, because afterwards is often too late. And if no teeth have appeared by your child's second birthday, she certainly needs a visit.

Teething

Babies are (with rare exceptions) born without teeth. When the milk teeth erupt will depend on your child, but her lower front teeth will usually be the first to appear, between six and nine months. By 15 months, she will have all her eight incisors, and the full set of 20 milk teeth will usually have surfaced by the time she is three years old.

HOW BABY TEETH GROW

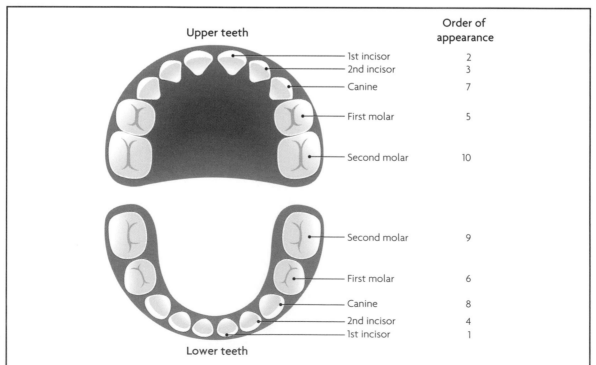

Upper teeth	Order of appearance
1st incisor	2
2nd incisor	3
Canine	7
First molar	5
Second molar	10
Second molar	9
First molar	6
Canine	8
2nd incisor	4
1st incisor	1

Lower teeth

Then the tooth fairy stage starts. She is likely to start losing her milk teeth when she is six, and they will keep dropping (to be replaced by permanent teeth) until she is around twelve. By the time she is finished, there will be 32 adult teeth. Both sets of teeth are very tough (the outer enamel is the hardest mineralised tissue in her body), but then they have to be.

Her milk teeth will need just as much care as her adult set. The outer enamel is thinner than that of permanent teeth, making them more vulnerable to decay as soon as they appear. If she loses any milk teeth too early, the other teeth will move and crowd the space, and there will be orthodontic visits in the future.

When your baby is teething, she will be grumpy but at most it will be moderately uncomfortable. You will see the tell-tale signs:

- Her cheeks will be red.
- She will drool more than usual.
- She will bite and chew anything in sight.
- Her nappies may be runnier than normal.

Home Treatment: Teething

Once the tooth breaks through her gum, all her teething problems will disappear. It is simply a question of time, but how can you ease things in the meantime?

Every family will have its own 'chewing' remedy for teething. You can try some of these:

- **Teething rings**
- **A cold spoon**
- **Frozen bread**
- **Teething gel**
- **A cold, wet facecloth**
- **Homeopathic granules.**

They will be a welcome distraction and she will like chewing them, though no studies have yet shown that chewing on something actually improves matters. Often, just rubbing her gum with your (clean) finger will help as the pressure alone can ease the pain. Teething biscuits are not a good idea, as they may contain sugar and they soften quickly. Try to avoid paracetamol if you can and never rub alcohol on a baby's gums.

A word of caution: teething does not give babies a high temperature, so if your child has one, look for another cause.

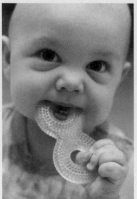

Teething ring

Accidents

If she falls and knocks out a tooth it is a dental emergency, especially if it is a permanent tooth. You need to put the permanent tooth back where it was quickly – ideally within one hour. The longer the delay, the less chance the tooth has of surviving.

Not so surprisingly, toddlers have the most accidents with teeth. And the teeth that suffer most are usually the middle incisors. You also need to watch your older child who plays contact sports. Without a mouth guard, she is six times more likely to damage her teeth. Custom-made mouth guards are best.

Home Treatment: Accidents

If a tooth falls out in an accident, visit your dentist as a matter of urgency.

But first:

- **If it is a permanent tooth**, wash it gently in clean water (to remove any debris) and put it back in the socket. Don't touch the root! Try to position it where it was.
- **If it will not go back**, store it in milk and bring it to your dentist.
- But if it is a milk tooth, **don't** replace it in the socket. It can affect the permanent tooth that is growing behind it. Let your dentist examine her.

There are live cells at the root of a tooth and they will help to heal it, but the cells die quickly so don't waste any time replacing a permanent tooth.

Decay and Erosion

Your child's teeth are vulnerable to decay from the moment they erupt, but luckily tooth decay is very preventable. Yet 50 per cent of children will have some decay before they are twelve. Sometimes the dental visit is too late and the only option is to extract the tooth. Where does it all go wrong?

It's mainly down to diet. Tooth decay is caused by disease (the bacterium *Streptococcus mutans*), but her diet will feed the problem. The bacteria break down any sucrose they find on her teeth and produce acids, which can destroy the tooth enamel by removing essential minerals. And because her defences are still immature, they can work faster.

Sugared drinks are the major cause of tooth decay (and this includes apparently healthy fruit juices and flavoured waters). The real problem is the child who has a bottle in her bed every night, filled with juice – the unpleasant results are what dentists call 'baby-bottle tooth decay'. Your child's teeth produce less saliva at night (leaving them more vulnerable) and if she falls asleep on a bottle of juice her teeth will soak in sugar/acid. But when she eats, she produces more saliva, which protects her teeth. So if she has to eat sugary drinks or foods, let it be at mealtimes. It also gives her saliva a clear working period between sugar attacks.

Erosion is just as much a problem as decay. While bacteria decay teeth, chemicals in the diet will wear away tooth enamel. The biggest culprit – once again – is juice and soft drinks. With older children, the problem is high-energy sports drinks and carbonated diet drinks. If your child drinks fruit juice more than once a day, she is three times more likely to have tooth erosion.

It's a sad fact that children who have tooth decay in their baby teeth are very likely to have decay in their adult teeth.

Home Treatment: Tooth Decay

You can prevent tooth decay or erosion:

- The **only** liquid in her bottle should be milk or water (never sugared drinks or fruit juice).
- **Don't let her sleep with a bottle** unless it contains water. And don't 'bottle prop' her milk feeds in her cot.
- **Stop using bottles during the day** after one year – teach her to use the cup instead.
- **Once her milk teeth appear,** brush them at least once a day. But don't use toothpaste until she is two years old.

- ✚ **Keep sugared drinks and fruit juices to the minimum** – and never between meals. They will not damage her teeth if she **only** drinks them at mealtimes. And using a straw will at least reduce contact with her teeth.

- ✚ **Encourage her to drink all drinks at once**, not in little sips.

- ✚ **Sweetened foods** should only be eaten with meals – not as snacks. And never as rewards. Some processed baby foods contain a lot of sugar, so check the contents.

- ✚ **Water** is the best drink between meals.

If she uses a soother, try to get rid of it by her first birthday. Otherwise your child will end up with crooked teeth.

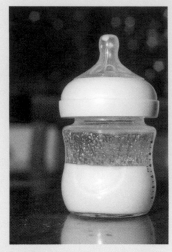

The only liquid in your child's bottle should be milk or water

Fluoride and Dental Sealants

Some people are uneasy about fluoride in public water supplies. Is it safe for your child? The best scientific evidence has found that fluoride levels at one part per million are perfectly safe, so reassure yourself by checking your local water authority's standard.

There is no doubt that fluoride will protect your child's teeth (look at the dental health of any population that uses it routinely in water). Fluoride is a mineral that is found naturally in rocks and soil. It is absorbed into the crystal of tooth enamel, making it less soluble and less likely to wear down. It also slows down bacterial fermentation of the sugar on teeth. In fact, getting the fluoride straight onto her teeth is even more effective – that is why we use fluoride toothpaste. You will not need fluoride tablets unless there is no fluoride in your local water (even if your baby is breastfed).

Fluorosis has become a little controversial, but it can be avoided and it is mainly a cosmetic problem. High doses of fluoride can lead to abnormal development of enamel on teeth and the result is white spots or blotches on the teeth. In fact up to 90 per cent of cases can only be seen by close dental examination.

Dental (fissure) sealants are one of the best protections your child's teeth can get and are recommended by every dental association. They prevent decay and cost one-third of the price of a tooth filling, so it is surprising that they are still under-used. While fluoride will protect the smooth surfaces of her teeth, a sealant keeps food out of the cracks and pits, where toothbrushes find it hard to reach. It's a plastic coating, which your dentist paints on her permanent teeth (usually the back chewing teeth, which are the most vulnerable) once they erupt. Sealants are safe and can reduce decay by 80 per cent in the two years after they are placed and they will continue protecting her teeth for up to ten years. They are strongly advised for your child.

APPLYING DENTAL SEALANT

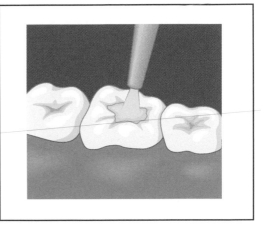

The dental sealant is painted on her teeth and hardens in seconds

Q&A

Q When should she first visit a dentist?

A Her first visit should be when her first tooth appears. This will probably be some time between six and twelve months old. As the American Academy of Pediatric Dentistry puts it: 'First visit by first birthday'. Problems can begin early and the biggest worry is always 'baby-bottle tooth decay'. It is also useful to get her used to the dentist's surgery when she is small so she is less likely to be scared later.

Q When should I start brushing her teeth?

A Her teeth must be kept clean as soon as they erupt, to prevent any decay, starting with her milk teeth. You can use a damp facecloth or a child's toothbrush, but don't use fluoride toothpaste until she is two years old. Always remember to brush the gums as well as the teeth, and don't overlook the backs of the teeth. It is also a good idea to floss gently, every few days or more if you can. Look out for spots on her teeth that are brown or chalk white as they may mean decay.

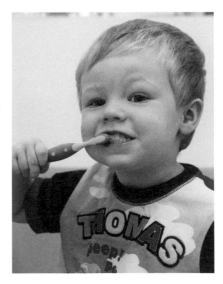

Q **What is plaque?**

A You brush her teeth twice a day to keep her gums healthy and to remove plaque. Plaque is a sticky white deposit that can build up on her teeth – it is a combination of food, saliva and millions of feeding bacteria. You remove it by brushing and flossing. But if you don't remove it, she is likely to get tooth decay or gum disease, or both. If you want to know how well you are dealing with plaque, try using a detector kit – it stains plaque deposits and shows you where you need to work at cleaning.

Saliva does wash plaque away and neutralise acids, but if your child's mouth is constantly bathed in sugar or acid (because of snacks) the saliva has little chance of doing its job.

Q **Why does she bleed when I brush her teeth?**

A Brush her teeth thoroughly, but not so hard that the gums bleed. If you are not a rough brusher, the bleeding could well be gingivitis, which is very common in children. Her gums will probably be blue/red and swollen but they will not hurt. If you use a plaque detector, you will see the cause of her problem – plaque deposits between her teeth. It comes from bad dental hygiene, so check her brushing. Are you using dental floss to get food out of the cracks?

Q **Why does she have some discoloured teeth?**

A Tooth staining is common enough in children and is often caused by bacteria in plaque. Better brushing usually solves the problem. But many foods (e.g. iron supplements) can also cause surface staining and if so your dentist can remove the stains. If your child has been quite ill recently (while her teeth were developing), it may have caused the discoloration. Or if she damaged a tooth in an accident, it may have turned black as a result. Sometimes excessive fluoride can be the problem (there's usually mild white discoloration) but it will not need any treatment. The antibiotic tetracycline is no longer used with children under eight years as their developing teeth absorb the drug and can change colour.

Section 3
Health Risks in the Pre-teen Years

WHAT TO LOOK OUT FOR IN EARLY ADOLESCENCE

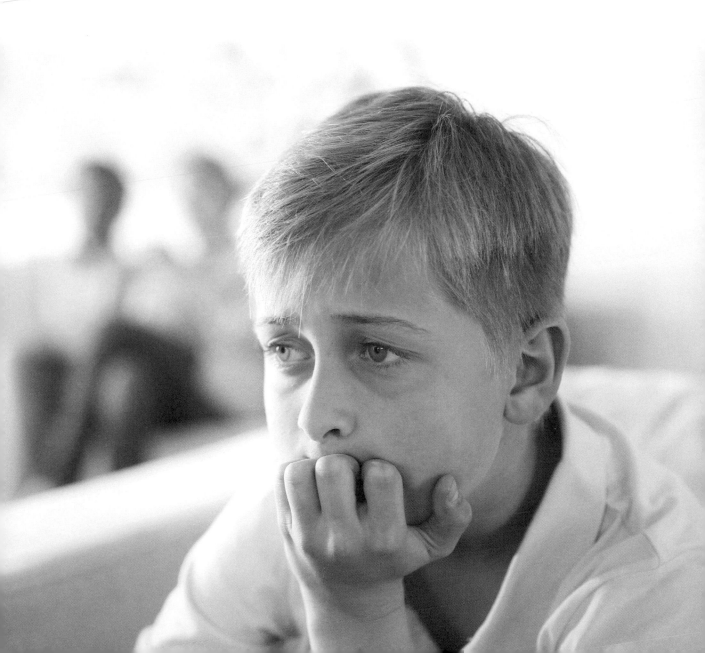

Chapter 25

Health Risks in the Pre-teen Years

Adolescence Starts Early

Just when you think that all the hard stages of child rearing are over, puberty starts to show and you have an adolescent. But these days your adolescent may not be a teenager. In fact, most children are now showing puberty changes between ten and twelve years old. This is a time of great personal change for your child, a physical process that affects her emotions – and potentially her health.

This chapter is not designed to alarm you. Luckily, most of the serious problems in these pages are not common, but they can creep up on a parent. And remember that, if they do, it will all happen much earlier than in your day. I am alerting you to certain health risks (and to the warning signs) as your child enters puberty. Hopefully you can prevent any problems setting in as a result.

Eating Disorders

If your child has an eating disorder it is not simply a 'phase' for attention seeking. She is ill, at great risk and needs immediate help. We see it more often in the mid-teens, but it can start before the age of twelve and I have seen cases (luckily rare) as young as nine. Puberty is the time when eating problems can begin. Your child is more insecure and for various reasons she can become dissatisfied with her changing body. Gradually, her self-worth becomes defined solely by how she (thinks she) looks.

She is most likely to have:

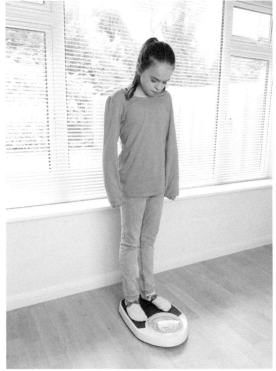

- 🧰 **Anorexia nervosa:** She is intensely scared of gaining weight, is unnaturally thin and has a distorted image of her own body.
- 🧰 **Bulimia nervosa:** She is caught up in a cycle. Out-of-control binge eating, followed by attempts to get rid of the food such as vomiting, using laxatives or over-exercising.

Nearly 2 per cent of girls are at risk. And the earlier a girl hits puberty, the more likely she is to develop an eating disorder. It is less common, but boys can also be affected. Sometimes the problem is not picked up because parents don't expect their son to have an eating problem. But it's not a 'girls' problem': both sexes can feel intense body dissatisfaction.

It's not always clear what causes a child to have an eating disorder. There may, in fact, be more than one reason. She may have a genetic tendency, which is triggered by puberty. She may be influenced by the impossible, 'thin' ideal in the media and – increasingly – by social media sites that promote dangerous 'skinny is perfect' messages. She may have low self-esteem or be a perfectionist. She may have a mother who diets – dieting mothers can lead to dieting daughters. It is less likely to be caused by a single incident.

What is certain is that children are learning unhealthy attitudes to their weight at an earlier age. Sadly, a study of five-year-old girls in the USA showed that many already associated 'diet' with restricting food. Another study of ten-year-olds showed that 81 per cent were afraid of being fat. And in the UK, national health guidelines on eating disorders now start with children aged eight. We are seeing large numbers of pre-teens caught up in weight anxiety and dieting is starting at a much younger age.

As a parent, you can help to prevent an eating disorder by being careful about the messages you give your child from a young age. Try to focus less on weight and appearance as important values (yours as well as hers), and more on personality. You can also usefully discuss media and social media images of the 'thin' ideal – and the reality – before she hits puberty. Steer her well away from the more extreme social media sites. And don't wait until she reaches her teens to promote a healthy body image.

Is It an Eating Disorder?

If you notice that your child's eating habits and mood have changed markedly, you need to talk to a professional. There can be early signs. Is she 'not hungry' at mealtimes, weighing herself several times a day and obsessed with food labels? We start to suspect an eating disorder if:

- She is 15 per cent below her expected weight for her age and height.
- She has intense fear of gaining weight (even if she is underweight).
- She has reached puberty but her periods stop (or puberty is delayed).
- She has a distorted image of her own body (I ask patients to draw a picture of themselves).
- She starts to wear layered or bulky clothes.
- She uses extreme methods to lose weight: self-induced vomiting, fasting, laxatives or excessive exercise.
- She becomes withdrawn.

Source: Based on the DSM-5 guidelines of the American Psychiatric Association, 2013.

When I examine her I am looking for an abnormally slow heart rate, marked weight loss, facial wasting and dull, thinning hair. Her hands and feet may be cold or swollen. I will carry out blood tests and an ECG and rule out other medical causes such as inflammatory bowel disease, coeliac disease, thyroid hormone problems and (something that is very rare) a tumour.

Will she be automatically admitted to hospital? No, unless it is an extreme situation. Most cases are treated as outpatients and research has shown this to be as effective as hospitalisation. But she will need medical and psychiatric help and I strongly advise the help of a family therapist too. Drug therapy is rarely needed. If your child has an eating disorder it will put great stress on your family and you will all need support in treating it. Her first step is to put on weight, but we also need to tackle her body image and her motivation for recovery.

Parents often worry that they are at fault, but it's important to know that they do not cause an eating disorder and are not to blame. I always try to focus less on why it happened and more on the solution. What I do stress is that an eating disorder has to be taken very seriously: she will not 'grow out of it' and without treatment it can be very dangerous. It is a chilling fact that 5 per cent of anorexics die and 20 per cent end up with eating disorders for life. So if you are concerned that your child may have an eating disorder, talk to your doctor immediately. Spotting the warning signs early is crucial. We know that young adolescents recover better if the problem is tackled promptly and if both parents and child can work together.

Post-viral Fatigue

Every early adolescent is tired. After all, growth is pretty wearing and so are the new demands of school and peers. But if your child is exhausted, despite good rest, and if routine medical tests have been negative, she may have post-viral fatigue.

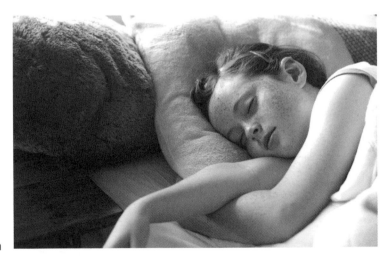

Young people do develop post-viral fatigue — also known as chronic fatigue syndrome or ME. With children, it usually appears from twelve to fourteen years, as they move into secondary school. But it can develop at an earlier age and the impact on your child's life can be quite dramatic. In fact it's the reason for nearly 40 per cent of all long-term absence from school in early adolescence. We are not certain what causes it, but it's believed that a viral infection may trigger the condition, especially when it is severe. And if a personal crisis or depression coincides with your child's infection, it may also help the fatigue to persist. Of course, if she pulls out of school and social activities because of illness she will feel quite isolated and this can make everything worse. But it's important to recognise that post-viral fatigue is a very real condition. It is not psychosomatic and it is not a veiled depression – it is a medical condition which has psychiatric aspects. In the past, it was known as the 'yuppie flu'; now we know that it can affect anyone. In fact it is more common in socially disadvantaged areas but is simply less likely to be diagnosed.

Parents in general are quite slow to seek help – only 31 per cent of children with post-viral fatigue will visit the doctor. But if you suspect it, it is very important to get help for your child. It can and it should be treated.

Is It Post-viral Fatigue?

Does she feel exhausted all the time? Has it lasted for more than three months and is it affecting relationships with her friends, her school attendance and her academic results? There is no test that proves that your child has post-viral fatigue and I will usually diagnose it based on symptoms. I look for a collection of them:

- Severe fatigue
- Headaches
- Poor concentration
- Depressed mood
- Poor sleeping patterns
- Muscle aches at rest and on exercise
- Poor appetite and nausea
- Joint pains.

Sometimes there is a weekly pattern of gradual fatigue. She goes to school on Monday, she is exhausted after sports on Wednesday and she misses school on Friday. It could, of course, be something else and I will always rule out another medical cause such as:

- Juvenile arthritis (she will have joint swelling and limited joint movement).
- Inflammatory bowel disease.
- Iron deficiency anaemia (a simple blood test will pick this up).
- Psychiatric illness such as anxiety disorder or depression (this may need a child or adolescent psychiatrist to make the diagnosis).
- Very rarely, a malignancy such as a brain tumour.

Treating post-viral fatigue is not straightforward and the condition is still not fully understood. If your child has it, she will be helped with a mixture of treatments but most likely:

- Cognitive behaviour therapy, to improve sleep quality and increase activity.
- Sleep routines, to avoid prolonged daytime sleeping, and relaxation exercises to wind down before sleeping. Melatonin may also be used to help with sleep issues.
- A very gradual increase in physical activity, with regular rest periods.
- Graded exercise therapy with a physiotherapist, to promote fitness and stamina.
- Pain management, generally with paracetamol or ibuprofen.
- School re-integration, starting with very short periods and gradually building up as tolerated. Home tuition may be needed.
- Some parents also use natural remedies. Relaxation therapies such as yoga can help, but herbal remedies and vitamin supplements do not seem to make any difference. St John's wort and comfrey can have toxic side effects.

Can you help prevent post-viral fatigue? Unfortunately, we still do not know enough about the condition to be clear. But as your child enters the pre-teen years, try to give her a healthy diet, to establish good sleeping and exercise habits and to avoid too many stresses in her daily life.

If she has post-viral fatigue and is treated promptly, the future is usually positive. Most early adolescents will make a full recovery within one to two years. Some will linger on and need continued medical support, because of ongoing symptoms.

Substance Abuse

Smoking Tobacco and E-cigarettes

If your child smokes tobacco, it will usually start in adolescence. If she starts, she will find it very hard to stop. She can be addicted to nicotine within a few months, so it is worth trying to prevent those first cigarettes. And, while there has been a fall-off in smoking generally, children are starting to smoke very young. The peak age for experimenting with cigarettes is now eleven to fifteen.

Most young smokers think that they can stop when they like. They don't understand, however, just how addictive nicotine is. In America, only 5 per cent of high school smokers believed that they would still be smoking after graduation. But five years later, 75 per cent were still smoking. Quitting is harder than they think.

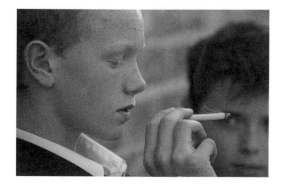

Cigarettes may not be the only problem, however. If your child smokes she may also open the door to other problems. She will be three times more likely than a non-smoker to use alcohol and eight times more likely to use cannabis. Researchers have also found a link between tobacco smoking in late childhood and depression as an adult. It really makes sense not to start in the first place. We all know, by now, the health consequences: above all, heart and lung damage and cancer.

Why do some people start smoking at a young age? A large study in New Zealand asked thirteen-year-olds this question. 'Image', it seems, was a more important reason for smoking at age eleven than at age thirteen. 'Friends' as a reason for smoking was consistent across age, while 'relaxation and pleasure' was even more consistent. Interestingly, 'health' as a reason **not** to smoke was not widely cited. Is the message about health damage not getting through?

Is Your Child Smoking Cigarettes?

It can be hard to spot if your pre-teen is smoking, but there are some warning signs:

- Do you smell smoke on her clothes or hair or in her room?
- Has she started using mouthwash or eating mints?
- Is her bedroom window often open?
- Have you found a cigarette or spent matches?

If you or your partner smokes, your child will be more likely to smoke too. If you stop smoking when your child is young, she is less likely to start later. But even more important are the smoking habits of your child's friends. They will, in fact, be the strongest influence on whether she takes up smoking.

You can reduce the chances of your child becoming a smoker:

- Start talking to her about smoking when she is six or seven and keep the conversation open.
- Be very clear that you don't want her to smoke.
- Teach her how to say 'no' when cigarettes are offered.
- Nobody smokes inside your house – not even visitors.
- Teach her how smoking harms nearly every organ of the body.
- Be very specific about the effects on her appearance: bad breath, smelly clothes, bad teeth, acne (and lots of wrinkles later).
- Know who her friends are and what they do together.
- Keep her busy with sports and other extra-curricular activities.
- If you smoke yourself, try to quit. And never let her have one of your cigarettes.

In 2012, the US Surgeon General gave some stark facts: of every three young smokers, only one will quit, and one of those remaining smokers will die from tobacco-related causes. So keep your child away from cigarettes, if at all possible. But if you do catch her smoking, it's better not to start a row and instead find out why. You can be practical about it. Look at the facts together: the effects on her body, looks, sports performance and cash reserves. If she finds it hard to give up cigarettes, you can get advice from your doctor or from a stop-smoking group for teens.

Despite their 'safer' image, e-cigarettes are not a harmless alternative. Tobacco companies are now investing heavily in a new billion-dollar industry – for good reason. In recent years, electronic smoking among US students has tripled and in 2014 nearly a quarter of sixteen- to seventeen-year-olds in Ireland had tried e-cigarettes. Yes, they contain less nicotine and fewer toxic substances than conventional tobacco. But despite marketing claims, opinion on whether they are actually safer is bitterly divided. They are still a very new, relatively untried product containing small amounts of carcinogenic chemicals. They may be better than smoking tobacco, but they are not harmless. And nicotine is very addictive. I'd advise keeping your child away from them too.

Alcohol

Alcohol abuse is perhaps a bigger risk for your child. Drinking is, after all, more socially acceptable, and some see it as a rite of passage. It is also easily available and can be cheap. What is worrying is the fact that drinking can start at a very young age. Fifty years ago, the average age in the USA for that first drink of alcohol was seventeen. In 2003, it was fourteen. Today, that figure has dropped even further in some countries.

I always advise parents to postpone that first drink as long as possible and, above all, to avoid under-age drinking. How your child comes to view alcohol is important. Before the age of nine, children generally see drinking alcohol as bad. By about age thirteen, however, their expectations shift and become more positive. In their teens they are quite likely to see drinking as central to their social life. Of course, this view will be reinforced if you, as a parent, drink considerably. Your attitude (despite what they tell you) does matter. Studies have shown that most teenagers believe that their parents should have a say in whether they drink alcohol. And if they know that their parents will be upset if they drink, they are less likely to do so. So it's up to you to have a consistent message. But remember that you have more influence on your child's attitude to alcohol **before** they take that first drink.

We know that the younger your child is when she starts drinking, the more likely she is to have alcohol problems in future life. She is also more prone to risky behaviour. And too much alcohol can have permanent effects on her developing young brain.

Is Your Child Drinking Alcohol?

Could your pre-teen be drinking? If she shows several of these signs at the same time or if they are very extreme, she could have a drinking problem:

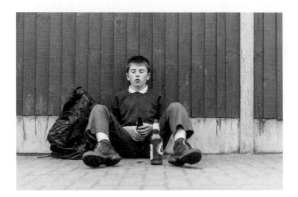

- Mood changes.
- Problems at school.
- Rebellion against family rules, and defensiveness.
- New friends who she's reluctant to introduce you to.
- Low energy and an 'I don't care' attitude.
- The smell of alcohol or alcohol hidden in her room.
- Bloodshot eyes and slurred speech.
- Loss of memory and poor concentration.

A child may start to drink alcohol for a variety of reasons and usually it coincides with puberty and new social pressures. But if she drinks too much, she will be stacking up serious medical problems for the future. Between 1995 and 2009, alcoholic liver disease rose by 275 per cent among fifteen- to 34-year-olds in Ireland. Alcohol doesn't only affect the body, however. Don't forget that it is a psychoactive, mood-changing drug. We may think it raises our spirits, but it is in fact a depressant. If your child drinks too much, she is very likely to develop depression problems too. And she will also be at a higher risk of injury. In the UK, a national survey of emergency departments found that 70 per cent of night-time cases were alcohol related.

How can you prevent your child from under-age drinking? It may not be easy, but your best tack is to set out clear rules against it and to be consistent in enforcing them. Try talking to your child from an early age about your concerns on alcohol and keep in touch with her friends' parents. Look for other parents who feel the same way about drinking (there will be more than you think) and create a united front. It's better not to provide alcohol at an under-age party (despite the protests) and never offer a drink to somebody else's child. Some parents will offer their child alcohol at home, to teach them to drink appropriately, and a sip of alcohol at a special family occasion is not out of place. But if your child is allowed to drink regularly at home she will drink more heavily outside the home.

The longer you can keep her away from alcohol, the better. But if you think, or know, that your child has a drink problem, you need to talk to her doctor or an alcoholism specialist. The biggest service you can give your child is to get help.

Drugs

Hopefully, your child will not use illegal drugs, but it does happen. In the UK, 7 per cent of eleven-year-olds and 31 per cent of fifteen-year-olds have taken drugs. Typically, younger children will try inhalants (using glue, petrol, spray paints or shoe polish to get a brief high), but they will also try sleeping pills and cannabis.

INHALANTS are often a child's first experience of drugs. Some even see them as 'kids' drugs' and somehow less harmful. Many children don't see them as drugs at all. After all, most of the products are part of everyday life, and children as young as five can quite easily discover the effects of inhaling them. But they are mind-altering drugs and they can be very dangerous. A child will breathe in chemical vapours for the high, but these chemicals can cause central nervous system damage, hearing loss and even heart attack. A single inhaling incident can kill – it's known medically as 'sudden sniffing death syndrome'. Could your child be playing around with inhalants? These can be signs of a problem:

- She seems to be drunk.
- She has sores around her nose or mouth.
- Her clothes smell of chemicals.
- Her breath is quite strange.

If you think she may be using inhalants, talk to her about the dangers and – if necessary – get specialist advice.

Then there are **SLEEPING PILLS**. A short dose is perfectly safe if your child has, for a very particular reason, bad insomnia. Perhaps exam anxiety or a family crisis. The problem is that regular use can make her dependent on the pills. Does she take them every time she feels anxious? Does she take them every night, just in case she can't sleep? There is also the problem of misuse. Sleeping pills are sedative hypnotics. Some young people mix them with alcohol, hoping to increase the effects of the high. And, very conveniently, they are more widely prescribed than before. No wonder that abuse of sleeping pills has risen in schools and colleges. My advice is to tread carefully when you consider giving sleeping pills to your child. Use them only for short-term, emergency situations. And hold on to that prescription (and supplies) yourself.

As for **CANNABIS**, it is now the most widely used illegal drug in Europe. It is also hotly debated: is it addictive or is it harmless? No, it is not harmless. It is, after all, a drug, and one that contains a mind-altering chemical known as THC. We know that, in recent times, higher levels of THC in the drug are making it more potent. We also know that it can cause problems with memory and affect school performance – a 2012 study even showed a connection between heavy cannabis use starting in the teens and a drop in IQ points. Not everybody will become addicted to it, but about one in six people who start using it in their teens will be. And now there is a new, more disturbing finding. It seems that using cannabis in your teens increases your chances of schizophrenia as an adult. If your child is regularly smoking cannabis, she will need help.

A final word of caution about **ECSTASY** (MDMA). It was barely known among adolescents in the early 1990s. Now it is a drug of adolescence – the 'party drug' - with its popularity waxing and waning over the years. Girls are more likely to use it than boys. It's a synthetic drug that energises (it has some of the same qualities as speed), but it also produces psychedelic effects. Ecstasy can be very dangerous as it affects the body's ability to control temperature. In extreme cases and in very hot situations, it can cause organ damage or even death. Your child is most likely to come across the drug in the mid-teen years – around fifteen or sixteen – but she may try it at a younger age. Whether she uses it or not will depend, to some extent, on how safe she thinks it is. Every time there is an ecstasy health scare, rates of usage drop quite significantly. So talk to her from an early age about the risks (and media reports of cases where it went badly wrong).

Is Your Child Using Drugs?

There are some red flags:

- Her friends have changed and she has not introduced them to you.
- Loss of interest in her personal appearance and things she used to enjoy.
- Sudden changes in mood.
- She has become more secretive.
- Missing school, sports or family events.
- A marked drop in her school grades.
- Increased requests for money or money going missing.
- Her appetite and sleeping habits have changed.
- You find cigarette papers, powders or tablets.

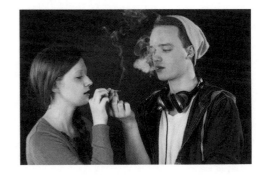

There has been much debate about the 'gateway theory': that cannabis and soft drug use leads to using addictive drugs like heroin. But experimenting with any drug is dangerous, especially if your child has a risk-taking or addictive personality. You need to have a very clear message around drugs, soft or hard: **don't**. If you suspect that she is taking drugs, you really need to talk to your doctor or a drug abuse clinic.

According to the National Center on Addiction and Substance Abuse at Columbia University, a child who reaches the age of 21 without smoking, using illicit drugs, or abusing alcohol is almost certainly never going to do so. That may be a tall order, but let's at least aim to keep our under-age children away from them.

Keeping Your Child Healthy and Well

FACTORS YOU SHOULD CONSIDER

Chapter 26

Natural Therapies & Your Child

A Patient-led Trend

Everyone wants what is best for their child and natural health products are often preferred on safety grounds. The options are now considerable and include the traditional medicines of China, India and North America. You can also treat your child with minerals, vitamins, homeopathy and other remedies based on plants or animals.

How many children are now using natural therapies? A recent national health survey in the USA found that 11 per cent of children had used complementary medicine and 1.8 per cent had used homeopathy in the previous year. This is low, if you compare it to adult use, and it may reflect some caution on the part of parents. Most of the children were using fish oils, melatonin, probiotics and chiropractic or osteopathic manipulation. These were most likely to be tried as remedies for colds, anxiety, neck pain, ADHD and sleep problems. But the survey also found that children with chronic illnesses are increasingly being given either complementary or alternative medicine – often at the same time as conventional drugs.

Worries about the safety of pharmaceutical drugs are largely behind this trend towards natural therapies. It is a patient-led trend and I sympathise with parents who are concerned and who try to make sense of the medical world. But any health product – whether pharmaceutical or natural – interferes with your child's body. **You need to be very sure why you are using it.**

Mainstream medicine is in a difficult position. It is slow to accept any health product until it has been tested as rigorously as the rest. But it is also wary of being labelled defensive, or even territorial. After all, as the 'traditional' health system in the West, it has long been the dominant voice. Of course, what is new to the West (complementary medicine) is seen as 'traditional' in other parts of the world. I am quite practical about it. Where a natural therapy has been shown in trials to be effective and safe, I recommend it. Otherwise, caution is advised.

How Do They Perform?

It is worth remembering that complementary and alternative medicine are not the same. Complementary medicine is used in addition to the standard care of your doctor. Used wisely, it can work for your child. I am less comfortable with any medicine that is a substitute. A useful first reference for parents might be the American websites Medline Plus (www.medlineplus.gov) or the National Center for Complementary and Integrative Health (www.nccih.nih.gov). These give very current information on natural products and evidence from controlled trials. Also useful is the Canadian Pediatric Complementary and Alternative Medicine Research and Education Network (www.pedcam.ca).

Some natural products have performed well in trials and there have been promising results. Cranberries have had some success in treating urinary tract infections in adults. Green tea seems, from preliminary trials, to help conditions such as arthritis and to prevent colds or flus – though it is still too early to be certain. The evidence for fish oil capsules in preventing heart disease is strong, despite earlier concerns about methyl mercury. And Asian ginseng appears to help the immune system and may lower glucose levels.

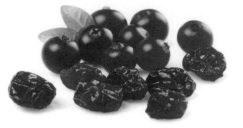

Cranberries have been used to successfully treat urinary tract infections in adults

Caution is advised, however, because many natural products have still to be tested as rigorously as conventional drugs. And, unfortunately, trial samples are often too small. While acupuncture can ease chronic pain in adults, there is still very little research on how it affects children. Calendula is commonly used for minor skin wounds, but most evidence for its wound-healing ability is based on animal research (there have been virtually no human studies yet). Where controlled trials have been carried out, some problems have emerged. St John's wort has been shown to help mild to moderate depression, but we also know that it can react dangerously with prescription drugs or other herbal remedies. The hormone melatonin is often used for sleep problems, but in children it can affect other hormones, especially around adolescence. And homeopathic remedies are presumed to be safe because they are highly diluted, but some products labelled as homeopathic contain high amounts of the ingredient. Like any drug, they can cause side effects.

The Canadian Pediatric Society gives some very sound advice about natural therapy products. Most sensible of all is applying standard medical 'first principles' in its advice to doctors and these are just as relevant to you when choosing a product for your child:

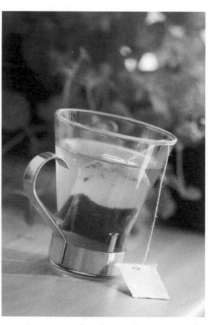

Green tea has been shown to help with arthritis and to prevent colds and flus

- ✚ First, do no harm.
- ✚ Don't delay treating a serious illness for which there is a **known** effective treatment.
- ✚ If the natural therapy has little risk of harm, consider using it and monitor it closely.
- ✚ If it carries serious risk of harm, warn the patient and monitor him closely.
- ✚ Where possible, use evidence-based decisions for a therapy.
- ✚ Where evidence is lacking, try to keep an open mind and a balanced approach.

It is worth bearing a few facts in mind:

- **Natural remedies are not tested as rigorously as pharmaceutical drugs.** If a product is labelled 'dietary supplement' it is not required to undergo the pre-market tests for safety and effectiveness that pharmaceutical drugs must pass. The label may also not reflect what is in the bottle.

- **Many natural remedies have not been tested for safety on children.** Few studies have examined the effects of complementary health products on children. Studies applied to adults can not automatically apply to children –the side effects can be very different.

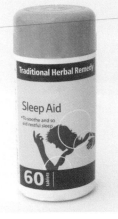

- **There is great variation in purity and strength.** Contamination is a concern: some Chinese medicines have caused heavy metal poisoning and a 2006 report by trading standard officers warned that these and herbal remedies can contain arsenic, mercury and asbestos.

- **The amount of active ingredient** across natural brands can range from 0 per cent to 200 per cent.

- **'The dose makes the poison.'** Children are not young adults. They are smaller, their bodies are still growing and immature and any drug, natural or conventional, will affect them differently (e.g. the immature blood-brain barrier in small babies can allow substances into the central nervous system). Less than 30 per cent of drugs approved by the US Food and Drug Administration are labelled for children too. Doses of any drug for children need to be cautious and given by someone who is formally trained in children's medicine.

- **The more drugs you take, the likelier you are to have an adverse reaction.** Parents often do not tell their doctor about natural remedies their child is taking, and mixing drugs can cause problems. Patients with serious or chronic illnesses are the most likely to use natural remedies as well as prescription medicine.

- **Pharmaceutical drugs are 'pure' versions of natural remedies.** Over a quarter of modern pharmaceutical drugs are based on plants. The rest are synthetically created in the laboratory. They are purified to distil only the beneficial substance so they are less likely to have harmful side effects.

- **The placebo effect is very powerful.** Many patients with minor illnesses (or self-healing viruses) will improve as a result of their belief that the drug is going to make them better.

My advice to parents is always:

- 🩹 **Don't assume that a 'natural' product is safer.** Look for objective, randomised controlled trials before you use it. Is the trial sample large enough to be valid? Is standard methodology used to interpret the results?

- 🩹 **Are you happy** that it is 'better' than a pharmaceutical drug?

- 🩹 **Don't mix drugs.** Tell your doctor if your child is taking any natural remedies. They may react with other drugs prescribed. And please tell her if there have been any bad reactions.

BUT

Remember that 'natural' is not a guarantee of safety.

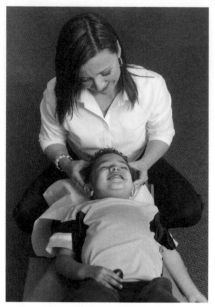

Chiropractic is a common complementing health approach.

TEN MOST COMMON COMPLEMENTARY HEALTH APPROACHES AMONG CHILDREN 2012

Natural products	
Dietary Supplements (other than vitamins and minerals)	4.9%
Chiropractic or Osteopathic Manipulation	3.3%
Yoga, Tai Chi, or Qi Gong	3.2%
Deep Breathing	2.7%
Homeopathy	1.8%
Meditation	1.6%
Special Diets	0.7%
Massage	0.7%
Guided Imagery	0.4%
Movement Therapies	0.4%

Source: L.I. Black, T.C. Clarke, P.M. Barnes, B.J. Stussman and R.L. Nahin, 'Use of complementary health approaches among children aged 4–17 years in the United States: National Health Interview Survey, 2007–2012', National Health Statistics Reports no. 78. Hyattsville, MD: National Center for Health Statistics, 2015.

Chapter 27

The Home Medicine Chest

Medical Supplies to Keep at Home

Your medicine cupboard does not have to be extensive, but there are some basics you are likely to stock for everyday – and home emergency – use.

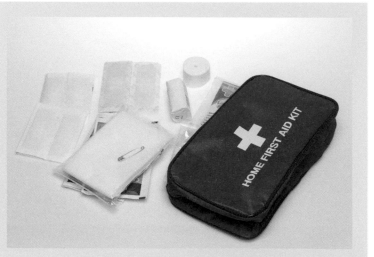

Paracetamol. Children's syrup and also tablets.

Ibuprofen. Children's syrup and also tablets.

Oral rehydration solution for stomach bugs (dehydration is a risk, especially with small children).

Thermometer. The type of thermometer is not as important as knowing how to use it (keep those instructions). If you use digital, have two thermometers in stock or keep spare batteries.

Antihistamines. Children's syrup but also tablets and cream. They reduce itching caused by allergies (such as hay fever), rashes and insect bites.

Calamine. Impregnated gauze or lotion. It soothes itchy skin caused by eczema, rashes and sunburn.

Decongestant capsules or tubes to ease blocked noses. If hay fever is a problem, keep oral decongestants during the peak season.

Antiseptic cream or solution for minor cuts.

Antifungal cream or powder for athlete's foot – especially in summer or for athletes in the house.

Emollients. Moisturising cream for dry skin.

Sun cream. Sun block is advised for children, which means any sunscreen with at least SPF 30 and UVA and UVB protection. Avoid sunscreen containing insect repellents.

Headlice treatment. A lice medication and special fine-toothed comb for 'bug busting' (if you start the treatment as soon as lice appear, you can avoid your child missing school).

Hydrocortisone cream for insect stings.

Barrier cream for nappy rash.

Plasters and bandages. Keep an assortment of plasters; it's also good to have a roll of crepe bandage with safety pins for injuries.

Sterile dressings for larger wounds.

Cotton wool. Keep it clean by storing it in a jar, or seal the opened bag.

Scissors and a tweezers for removing splinters or thorns.

Cough medicines are **not needed**, as there really is no evidence that they work.

Safety Policies

I advise four safety policies when it comes to medicines:

- Keep them high enough to be out of the reach of a toddler standing on a counter.
- Have a child lock on the cupboard door.
- Don't keep medicines that are out of date.
- Always read (and keep!) the instructions.

Chapter 28

'Is it Measles?' The Diseases Made Rare by Vaccination

Rare, But They Do Happen

Thanks to vaccination, these diseases are no longer common. But if you suspect that your child is infected, make sure to check it out.

Look for the symptoms.

Measles

- It starts with a runny nose, headache and cough.
- The temperature can be high and last at least four days.
- You will see tiny white spots inside the mouth and cheeks.
- The eyes will be red and sore.
- Then the flat, red/brown rash appears. First behind the ears, then on the face and body.
- The spots are separate at first, then they blend together to make the skin look blotchy.

The problem with measles is that complications can develop. For example, 1 in 25 people will get pneumonia; 1 in 1,000 will get encephalitis.

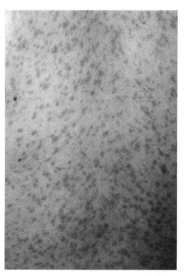
Measles

Mumps

- It starts with a temperature, a headache and a dry mouth.
- Then the glands under the chin swell and become sore – the face becomes puffy on one or both sides. It hurts when your child swallows.
- If he's a boy, his testicles may be sore and swollen.

Mumps can have serious complications, especially affecting the testes in boys. Before vaccination, it was one of the main causes of nerve deafness in children.

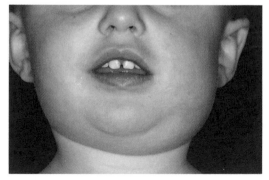
Mumps

Whooping Cough (Pertussis)

- It starts like a cold, with a cough, a runny nose and a slight temperature.
- Then the whooping begins. There will be long bouts of coughing followed by a 'whooping' sound and it will usually make him vomit. There will be pauses in breathing for several seconds.

It is a prolonged and distressing illness and the most serious effects are in babies under six months old.

Meningitis

- Fever.
- A flat, spotty rash that does not fade when pressed.
- Unusual drowsiness.
- Unusual crying.
- Vomiting.
- Cold hands and feet, leg pains and skin colour change.
- (In older children) headache, stiff neck, cannot tolerate bright light.

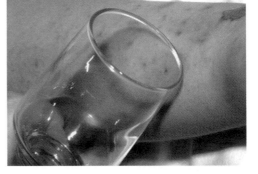

Meningitis

A meningitis rash has flat spots that **don't fade** when you press the base of a drinking glass against them. But sometimes there's no rash at all. If your child has **a number of these symptoms**, you should call your doctor or hospital at once.

Rubella (German Measles)

- There may be a slight temperature.
- A rash of tiny pink or red spots appears, first behind the ears, then it spreads to the forehead and finally the rest of the body.
- The spots merge as the rash spreads.
- The glands behind the neck will be swollen.

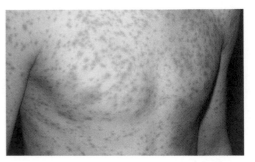

Rubella

The biggest problem is the devastating effects on an unborn child if a pregnant mother catches it. The virus will cause serious birth defects. The vaccine is an important protection.

Contact your doctor at once if you think your child may be infected. Don't call to the surgery – phone first.

Chapter 29

The Vaccine Debate

Do You Vaccinate Your Child?

When the time comes – it usually starts with the 6-in-1 vaccination – it's a tough question for any parent. Do I vaccinate? What makes it harder are the media scares about vaccines that went wrong. The facts are perhaps a little less exciting, but they are backed up by every reputable scientific body.

Yes, vaccinate your child.

- If she gets any of the 'vaccine' diseases, there is a risk of serious complications – even death.
- These risks are much, much higher than any problem a vaccine can cause.
- You cannot 'just put her on antibiotics' if she gets infected.
- Vaccinations have saved millions of lives since they were first introduced. They have virtually wiped out diseases that once haunted our world.
- Some of these diseases are now creeping back because of the drop in vaccinations. Vaccines will protect her.

If you pinned your doctor to the wall with the ultimate question – 'Would you vaccinate if it was your child?' – the answer would be the same: Yes.

How Vaccination Works

It is not quite homeopathy, but it is similar. Your child is given a tiny dose of the disease (all or part of a micro-organism that causes it) and her body goes into immune response mode. It fights back as if it were fully infected, but with little or no risk to your child. It's artificial immunity, but it works and it's far safer than natural immunity.

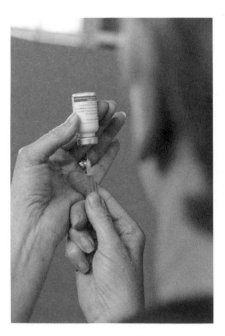

Some vaccines are now well established; others are more recent. New vaccines that may well be introduced in your country include the rotavirus vaccine against gastroenteritis, the varicella vaccine against chickenpox and the meningococcal b vaccine.

THE EFFECT OF VACCINATION ON ANNUAL CASES OF PREVIOUSLY 'COMMON' DISEASES

Disease	Average annual cases	Cases 1998 (after vaccination)	% decrease (20th century)
Smallpox	48,164	0	100
Diphtheria	175,885	1	100
Whooping cough	147,271	7,405	95
Tetanus	1,314	41	97
Polio	16,316	1	100*
Measles	503,282	100	100*
Mumps	152,209	666	>99
Rubella	47,745	364	>99

* Rounded to the nearest tenth

Source: Red Book 2000, Report of the Committee on Infectious Diseases, American Academy of Pediatrics.

Why Some Parents Don't

Q&A

Q Most of these diseases have been wiped out already – so why bother?

A In fact, they have not been wiped out. They have simply been reduced to near pulp because of vaccination programmes. But in any country, the 'safety boundary' is over 95 per cent of people vaccinated. At that level you have population immunity. Anything less than that means the disease can creep back. Many countries are near, or at, that boundary of safety already. It's a bit alarming when there are outbreaks in different parts of Europe and they are rising. Russia had one of the most disturbing in recent times, when a diphtheria epidemic broke out in 1993. It was disturbing because diphtheria is practically unheard of in the West.

Always remember that, apart from the smallpox virus, the germs are still out there. And when you have an outbreak, the safest state to be is vaccinated.

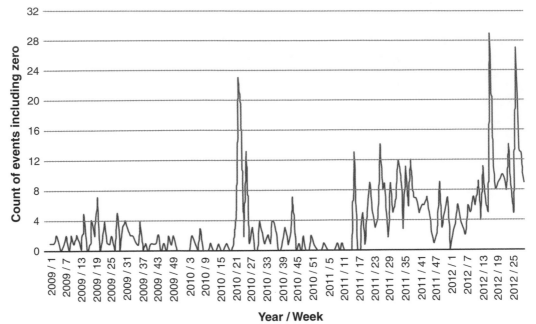

WHOOPING COUGH CASES REPORTED IN IRELAND 2009–2012

A rise in whooping cough in babies is a particular worry.

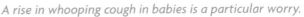

Q **You might get a bad batch of vaccines.**

A There really is no evidence that single batches of vaccines vary in safety. All vaccines are licensed and checked both before and after they are released.

Q **It's dangerous to give a baby a multiple vaccine all in one go.**

A The whole point of vaccines is to strengthen a baby's immune system – not to weaken it. There are 24 different antigens in the MMR vaccine. This is minute if you compare it to the number of antigens her immune system is able to deal with – up to 100 billion. They've studied the immunisation programme in great detail, especially the 6-in-1 vaccine. Every study has shown that it works and is safe. It gives your child immunity from the earliest possible stage and combining the vaccinations in one dose means less trauma for her.

Nowhere in the world are separate vaccines recommended. In Japan they give single vaccinations for measles and rubella and no mumps vaccine – but they have had a rise in deaths from measles.

Q You don't need vaccines – better living conditions got rid of most of these diseases.

A You will hear this said frequently. Of course, better living conditions have hugely reduced the spread of diseases. But they have not got rid of diseases – vaccination has. The Hib vaccine is a good example. Hib disease was a problem until recent years, in spite of modern living standards, but since the vaccination started it has virtually disappeared.

Russia's major epidemic of diphtheria was not because living conditions had disimproved (they hadn't), but because vaccination rates were low.

Q Most people who actually get these diseases have been vaccinated.

A It's true. When there's an outbreak, those who have been vaccinated often outnumber those who have not. If you think about, it makes sense. In developed countries, the majority of people will have been vaccinated and a tiny percentage will not have developed immunity. That's because vaccines are weakened to be safer than the disease. No vaccine is 100 per cent foolproof, but they are still the best possible protection for your child.

But in an outbreak, the vaccinated person will tend to get a milder form of the disease and vaccine failure is rare once a child has had two doses.

Q The MMR vaccine can cause serious problems. There's autism, for a start, and Crohn's disease.

A Very rarely, the MMR vaccine can cause serious after-effects. But studies in 1999 linking it to autism and Crohn's disease have now been discredited.

Worries about a link began with a hypothesis (by Dr Wakefield at the Royal Free Hospital in London) that MMR immunisation might be related to autism. But no study since then (and it has now been investigated to within an inch of its life) has found a connection. The largest study, published in 2015, analysed more than 95,000 children who did, and did not, get the MMR vaccine. Not only did the study find no link between the MMR vaccine and autism; it also found no link even in 'high-risk' families, where there was an older child with autism. The medical world now accepts that the MMR vaccine does **not** cause autism.

In 1993 Dr Wakefield also suggested a link to Crohn's disease because the measles virus seemed to be in the gut of patients with Crohn's disease. But after more sensitive tests, Dr Wakefield later confirmed that there was no measles virus in patients with the disease. There have been larger trials since then and they have shown that there's **no** link between Crohn's disease and the MMR vaccination.

The **actual** risks attached to the MMR vaccine are:

+ 1 in 1,000 may have fever fits.

+ Fewer than 1 in 10,000 may develop meningitis.

+ 1 in 22,000 can develop ITP (low blood platelets).

+ 1 in 100,000 can have an anaphylactic shock reaction.

Is this a reason not to vaccinate? Not when you remember that she's much more likely to get these problems if she catches the disease. For example, if she gets measles or mumps the chances of getting meningitis rise to 1 in 1,000. If she gets measles, the risks of death are 1 or 2 in 1,000. Nobody dies from a vaccine.

The MMR vaccination has been used for over 30 years now. Before it was first licensed, it was rigorously tested. Now, after decades of experience and studies, the World Health Organization has confirmed that it's one of the safest vaccines ever produced. After 500 million doses worldwide, it has proved itself – you cannot get a better trial than that.

And there is no increased risk from a second dose of the MMR vaccine (apart from an allergic reaction).

Q The whooping cough vaccine can cause permanent brain damage.

A In the 1970s the vaccine got a bad name because of reports that children had suffered brain damage and other problems after vaccination. When researchers investigated, however (and the studies were very detailed), they found that the claims did not hold up. There is, in fact, no evidence that the vaccine causes brain damage. Any risks associated with whooping cough vaccine are remote. The risks associated with getting the disease (including brain damage) are far, far higher.

Q I'm confused. Is it a 6-in-1 or a 3-in-1 injection?

A There is now a 6-in-1 vaccination to protect your child from six very serious diseases: diphtheria, whooping cough, tetanus, Hib (haemophilus influenzae b), polio and pneumococcal disease. The 3-in-1 is gone.

One dose is not enough to make her immune. She will get the 6-in-1 three times while she's a child – before her first birthday. At the same time, she will also get another vaccination to protect her against meningococcus C disease. Vaccine policy varies from country to country.

Q I don't like injecting anything into my child so young. Why do they give the MMR vaccine at 15 months.

A More than likely, your child had antibodies in her body when she was born. She had them because her mother was most likely vaccinated against the MMR diseases – or caught the infection at some stage. The antibodies remained in the mother's blood and were naturally passed on to the baby, giving immunity. But between six and 12 months, the antibodies (and immunity) decline. If we vaccinate earlier – into blood that already has the antibodies – the vaccine will be effectively inactivated.

Q If no one else is vaccinating, why should she? Isn't she likely to get it anyway?

A If you want to protect your child, vaccinate her. Most people in developed countries still get vaccinated (over 90 per cent in most EU countries), but some countries have slipped below the 'safety boundary'. Without a vaccine, she is more vulnerable.

What Will Happen if We Stop Vaccinating Children?

This generation has been very fortunate. Few people will witness the terrible effects of diseases such as measles and whooping cough – when they go badly wrong. Unfortunately, in our hospitals we still see children who suffer very badly, and even die, because their parents have not vaccinated them.

- A child with measles has a 1 in 10 chance of ending up in hospital.
- Mumps is one of the most common causes of deafness in children.
- Rubella is very dangerous to unborn children. It can cause serious disability and heart defects.
- 80 per cent of children who are not vaccinated will get whooping cough.
- In the developing world (where vaccination is scarce) 1 in 5 children can die before their first birthday from these diseases.

If you are really interested in scaring yourself, look up some old medical photographs. See the polio wards where children spent years lying in iron lungs. See babies born totally rigid with lockjaw. See children suffocating from diphtheria and others dying of brain degeneration because of measles.

Always remember that the germs haven't gone away. They are still out there.

Useful References &
Further Reading

Medical journals are among the best sources of current medical research and thinking on children's illness. But I hope that the selection of books and websites in these pages will be useful.

GENERAL

Cochrane Library (healthcare databases) – www.thecochranelibrary.com

Great Ormond Street Hospital, *New Baby and Child Care Book*, Random House, 2010

Medscape (web-based medical information for health professionals) – www.medscape.com

O'Neill, Michael, Michelle Mary McEvoy and Alf J. Nicholson, *Diagnosing and Treating Common Problems in Paediatrics*, Radcliffe Publishing, 2014

Stoppard, Miriam, *Complete Baby and Child Healthcare*, Dorling Kindersley, 2001

UpToDate (electronic updates for the medical community on the latest medical findings) – www. uptodate.com

Van Dorp, F. and C. Simon, *Child Health*, Oxford General Practice Library, 2007

CHAPTER 1 ASTHMA

American Academy of Allergy, Asthma and Immunology – www.aaaai.org

British Thoracic Society 'British Guidelines on the Management of Asthma, 2014 – www.brit-thoracic.org.uk

European Academy of Allergy and Clinical Immunology – www.eaaci.org

National Heart, Lung and Blood Institute, *Guidelines for the Diagnosis and Management of Asthma*, 2007 – www.nhlbi.nih.gov

Welch, Michael J., *Allergies and Asthma: What Every Parent Needs to Know*, American Academy of Pediatrics, 2010.

CHAPTER 3 CHEST INFECTION

American Academy of Pediatrics, *Diagnosis and Management of Bronchiolitis*, 2015 update – www. aap.org

Scottish Intercollegiate Guidelines Network, *Bronchiolitis in Children*, 2006 – www.sign.ac.uk
UpToDate, 'Bronchiolitis in Infants and Children', 2015 - www.uptodate.com

CHAPTER 4 **CONSTIPATION**

Bracey, Jackie, *Solving Children's Soiling Problems*, Churchill Livingstone, 2002

Clayden, Graham and Ulfur Agnarsson, *Constipation in Childhood*, Oxford University Press, 1991

National Collaborating Centre for Women's and Children's Health, *Constipation in Children and Young People*, RCOG Press, 2010

CHAPTER 5 **ECZEMA**

American College of Allergy, Asthma and Immunology – www.acaai.org

Cochrane Skin Group (UK) – www.skin.cochrane.org

National Eczema Society (UK) – www.eczema.org

National Institute for Health and Clinical Excellence (UK) – www.nice.org.uk

CHAPTER 7 **FEEDING PROBLEMS**

Dunne, T., P. Farrell and V. Kelly, *Feed Your Child Well*, Children's University Hospital, Temple Street, Dublin and A & A Farmar, 2008

Lawrence, Ruth A., *Breastfeeding: A Guide for the Medical Professional*, Elsevier Health Sciences, 2011

Spencer, Andy and Liz Jones, 'Understanding Breastfeeding: How to Offer Practical Help', *Current Paediatrics*, 2002, 12: 93–7

CHAPTER 9 **FITS & FAINTS**

Epilepsy Action – www.epilepsy.org.uk

Epilepsy Foundation – www.epilepsy.com

Epilepsy Ireland – www.epilepsy.ie

CHAPTER 10 **FOOD ALLERGY**

European Academy of Allergy and Clinical Immunology – www.eaaci.org

EuroPrevall, *Outpatient Clinic Study on Food Allergy*, 2015

Irish Food Allergy Network – www. ifan.ie

Jackson, Mark, *Allergy: The History of a Modern Malady*', Reaktion Books, 2006

Prescott, Susan L., *et al.*, 'A Global Survey of Changing Patterns of Food Allergy Burden in Children, *World Allergy Organisation Journal*, 2013 – www.waojournal.org

CHAPTER 20 **WATERWORKS & WETTING PROBLEMS**

American Academy of Family Physicians – www.aafp.org

Medline Plus (a service of the US National Library of Medicine and the National Institutes of Health) – www.medlineplus.gov

National Institute for Health and Clinical Excellence (UK) – www.nice.org.uk

CHAPTER 22 **THE NORMAL STAGES OF DEVELOPMENT**

Feigelman, S. 'The Preschool Years' in R.M. Kliegman, R.E. Behrman, H.B. Jenson and B.F. Stanton (eds), *Nelson Textbook of Pediatrics*

Sharma, Ajay and Helen Cockerill, *Mary Sheridan's From Birth to Five Years: Children's Developmental Progress*, Routledge, 2014

Sheridan, Mary D., *From Birth to Five Years*, Routledge, reprinted 2003

CHAPTER 24 **HOW TO GROW NORMAL TEETH**

American Academy of Pediatric Dentistry – www.aapd.org

British Dental Association – www.bda.org

Dental Health Foundation (Ireland) – www.dentalhealth.ie

CHAPTER 25 **HEALTH RISKS IN THE PRE-TEEN YEARS**

Academy for Eating Disorders, *AED Medical Risk Management Handbook*, 2011

Action on Smoking and Health (ASH), 'How smoking affects the way you look' – www.ash.org.uk

Bryant-Waugh, Rachel and Brian Lask, *Eating Disorders: A Parents' Guide* (2nd edn), Routledge, 2013

Cool Spot: a website on alcohol abuse developed specifically for children aged 11 to 13 – www. thecoolspot.gov

Healthy Teen Project – www.healthyteenproject.com

Muisener, Philip P., *Understanding and Treating Adolescent Substance Abuse*, Sage, 1994

National Health Service (UK), 'How will smoking affect your appearance?', a video about smoking and appearance designed for girls – www.nhs.uk/Video/Pages/Smokingmakeover

Neumark-Sztainer, D., *I'm Like, So Fat*, Guildford Press, 2005

Psych Central, useful tips for parents to help teens with drug problems – www.psychcentral.com.

Substance Abuse and Mental Health Services Administration (USA) – www.samhsa.gov

Viner, Russell (ed.), *ABC of Adolescence*, Wiley, 2013

CHAPTER 26 **NATURAL THERAPIES & YOUR CHILD**

Centers for Disease Control and Prevention, National Center for Health Statistics (USA), *National Health Interview Survey, 1997–2012*

Medline Plus, a service of the US National Library of Medicine and the National Institutes of Health – www.medlineplus.gov

National Center for Complementary and Inegrative Health (USA) – www.nccih.nih.gov

Pediatric Complementary and Alternative Medicine Research and Education Network (Canada) – www.pedcam.ca

CHAPTER 29 **THE VACCINE DEBATE**

Centers for Disease Control and Prevention (USA), information about the safety of specific vaccines – www.cdc.gov/vaccinesafety

National Disease Surveillance Centre (Ireland): www.ndsc.ie

Index